NEUROSCIENCE RESEARCH PROGRESS

DEVELOPMENT OF THE CEREBELLUM

CLINICAL AND MOLECULAR PERSPECTIVES

NEUROSCIENCE RESEARCH PROGRESS

Additional books and e-books in this series can be found on Nova's website under the Series tab.

NEUROSCIENCE RESEARCH PROGRESS

DEVELOPMENT OF THE CEREBELLUM

CLINICAL AND MOLECULAR PERSPECTIVES

SEVERINA FABBRI
EDITOR

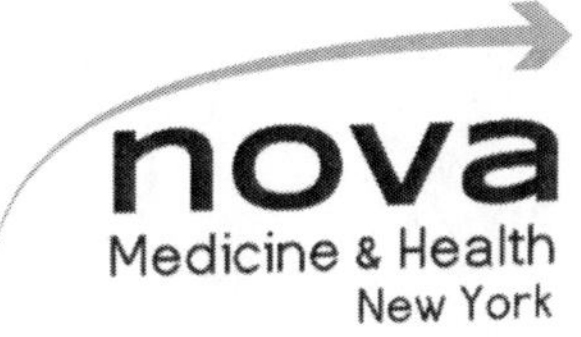

Library of Congress Cataloging-in-Publication Data

ISBN: 978-1-53614-317-1

Published by Nova Science Publishers, Inc. † New York

CONTENTS

PREFACE

The cerebellum is an important part of the central nervous system in most vertebrates. This brain structure is involved in several functions, such as motor control, reflex adaptation, motor learning and cognition (Buckner 2013; Lupo et al., 2018). The opening review in this compilation focuses on the development of the cerebellum, and more specifically, on the production of several types of neurons. It will show that these cells are sequentially generated following strict neurogenetic timetables.

Following this, the authors review manuscripts focusing on the negative impacts of maternal diabetes in pregnancy on the developing cerebellar cortex. Dissecting out the mechanisms responsible for maternal diabetes-related changes in the development of cerebellum is helpful in preventing impaired neurocognitive and neurobehavioral functions in offspring. The authors also investigate the consequences of repetitive drug administration on cerebellar synaptic efficiency. Insight into the neural mechanisms underlying these impairments has largely stemmed from clinical animal studies. The molecular and neuronal actions of addictive drugs in the cerebellum involve long-term adaptive changes in receptors, neurotransmitters and intracellular signaling transduction pathways that may lead to the reorganization of cerebellar microcomplexes or recreation of new domains of attraction. The gecko is proposed as a prospective animal model for a spaceflight experiment. Geckos demonstrate effective adaptation to weightlessness, quickly attaching themselves to surfaces by means of their subdigital pads, and during the spaceflight they retain both attached positions and normal locomotion, showing normal foraging, exploratory, social, and even play behavior. The role of cerebellum in geckos' adaptability to spaceflight and morphological changes in the cerebellum under the influence of microgravity are discussed. Next, an investigation was performed on Wistar rats with STZ – induced (60.0 mg/kg, i.p.) diabetes. High frequency (100 Hz) were delivered to VI-th lobula of paleocerebellum in two different regimes – one ES per two daily and thrice per day. VEP were registered in 6 and 12 weeks from the moment of diabetes induction. Lastly, a meta-analysis of recent findings of cerebellar involvement in executive functions in the elderly is provided. A methodological issue is raised which is relevant for models explaining cerebellar connectivity and effects on cognitive performance in old age.

Chapter 1 - The cerebellum is a region of the vertebrate nervous system involved in functions such as motor coordination, perception, cognition and development of the language. The anatomical structure of the adult cerebellum consists of a three-layered cortex and a set of cerebellar nuclei embedded in the white matter. There is evidence indicating that the germinal source of cerebellar neurons is heterogeneous. GABAergic neurons, such as inhibitory interneurons and some deep neurons, originate from the cerebellar neuroepithelium. On the other hand, glutamatergic neurons, including deep cerebellar nuclei neurons and unipolar brush cells, arise from progenitors located in the anterior rhombic lip. Granule cell precursors also originate from the rhombic lip and migrate tangentially over the surface of the cerebellar anlage to form the external granular layer. As indicators of DNA synthesis, tritiated thymidine and 5-bromo-2´-deoxyuridine have shown that one of the most important features of the cerebellar development is that each neuronal population is generated during a specific temporal window. This is named timetable of neurogenesis or time of neuron origin. It allows for an accurate delineation of both the onset and cessation of neurogenesis as well as for the determination of the proportion of neurons that are produced during single days of embryonic or postnatal life. The authors will show here that several types of cerebellar neurons are generated sequentially: first, the output neurons (deep neurons and Purkinje cells) and then, the interneurons (Golgi, unipolar brush, basket, stellate and granule cells).

Chapter 2 - There is increasing evidence that maternal diabetes mellitus during the pregnancy period is associated with a higher risk of neurodevelopmental and neurofunctional anomalies including motor dysfunctions, learning deficits, and behavioral problems in offspring. The cerebellum is a part of the brain that has long been recognized as a center of movement balance and motor coordination. Moreover, recent studies in humans and animals have also implicated the cerebellum in cognitive processing, sensory discrimination, attention, and learning and memory. Nevertheless the exact mechanisms by which maternal diabetes in pregnancy influence the development of the cerebellum are unclear and further study will be necessary to define the reason for these abnormalities observed in children born to diabetic women. Results from previous studies demonstrated that multiple biological alterations occur in pregnancies with diabetes and affect the development of fetal central nervous system (CNS), including in uterus hyperglycemia and hyperinsulinemia, neonatal hypoglycemia, and oxidative stress. Recent researches have clearly established that maternal diabetes disrupts the expression of insulin and insulin-like growth factor-1 receptors in the cerebellum of rat newborn. There is also evidence indicating that diabetes in pregnancy disrupts the synaptogenesis in the developing cerebellum. Here, the authors review the manuscripts focusing on the negative impacts of maternal diabetes in pregnancy on the developing cerebellar cortex. Dissecting out the mechanisms responsible for maternal diabetes-related changes in the development of cerebellum is helping to prevent from impaired neurocognitive and neurobehavioral functions in offspring.

Chapter 3 - Acute and chronic opioid consumption causes significant impairments in motor functioning, suggest an involvement of cerebellar circuits in fine tuning of movement patterns. Increasing evidence has involved the cerebellum in addictive behavior. The authors aimed on cellular and molecular targets in the cerebellum where opioids can induce or alter mechanisms of neuroplasticity that may contribute to the development of an addictive behavioral pattern. Also, the authors investigated the consequences of repetitive drug administration on cerebellar synaptic efficiency. Insight into the neural mechanisms underlying these impairments has largely stemmed from clinical animal studies. The results of these studies agree to relevant participation of the cerebellum in the functional systems underlying drug-induced long-term memory and the perseverative behavioral phenotype. The molecular and neuronal actions of addictive drugs in the cerebellum involve long-term adaptive changes in receptors, neurotransmitters and intracellular signaling transduction pathways that may lead to the reorganization of cerebellar micro complexes or recreation of new domains of attraction. As a part of this functional reorganization, drug-induced cerebellar hyper-responsiveness appears to be central in reducing the influence of executive control of the prefrontal cortex on behavior and aiding the transition to an automatic mode of control. As a result, it can be expected that improved understanding of the neural mechanisms affected by drug addiction has the potential to advance the diagnoses, treatment or even prevention of behavioral disorders.

Chapter 4 - In humans and other vertebrates, alterations in vestibular and motor function, including changes in linear vestibular-ocular reflexes, postural control systems, and so on, have been described under spaceflight conditions. Cerebellar structures are proposed to be involved in vestibular and locomotor disturbances in weightlessness. The gecko (*Chondrodactylus turneri* GRAY 1864) is a prospective animal model for a spaceflight experiment. Geckos demonstrate effective adaptation to weightlessness, quickly attaching themselves to surfaces by means of their subdigital pads, and during the spaceflight they retain both attached positions and normal locomotion, showing normal foraging, exploratory, social, and even play behavior. The cerebella of the thick-toed geckos after a 30-day spaceflight aboard "Bion-M1" biosatellite were examined and compared with terrarium and delayed synchronous control groups. Immunohistochemical and classical histological methods were used to reveal cell types in the anterior and posterior (vestibular) cerebellum. In general, the histological appearance of the cerebellum was normal in all groups of geckos. However, some pathomorphological changes in the Purkinje cells (such as chromatolysis, vacuolization, and hyperchromatosis) were detected. These cytomorphological features are a manifestation of the *in vivo* state of neurons, which correlates with the level of metabolism. A significant increase in the number of Purkinje cells with such changes were revealed only in the posterior vestibular cerebella of the geckos from the flight group in comparison with the control groups. It is reasonable to speculate that these changes detected in vestibular cerebellum Purkinje cells of geckos were caused by functional loading on the cells of this type during the spaceflight. Similar data were obtained during the Purkinje cell study using neuron-specific beta-III-tubulin (NST) immunohistochemistry. Immunoreactivity to NST was heterogeneous (decreasing in some cases and increasing in others) in Purkinje cells of the vestibular cerebellum of animals from all groups. An increase in the number of Purkinje cells with an altered NST immunoreactivity was revealed in the flight group. The authors did not identify any significant differences in the distribution and NST immunoreactivity of Purkinje cells in anterior cerebellum between flight and control groups of geckos. The density of Purkinje cell dendrites was also measured in the molecular layer of the anterior and posterior cerebellum. There were no statistically significant alterations of the dendrite density between groups both in the anterior and posterior cerebellum. The data coincide with the gecko behavior during the spaceflight, which was described in the "Bion-M1" space mission project. The authors propose that the nervous system is able to compensate for incorrect information from the vestibular system, using tactile and visual signals. The gecko is a prospective animal model to enable study of the cerebellum of vertebrates after a spaceflight due to the relative simplicity of its organization and, at the same time, its similarities with other vertebrates.

Chapter 5 - *Introduction:* Diabetes deteriorates visual pathway functioning, which manifests as a longer visual evoked potential (VEP) latency and reduced wave amplitude. These deteriorations indicate retinopathy development, which is severe and resistant to diabetes treatment. Cerebellar electrical stimulation (ES) does not directly affect VEPs. However, possible curative effects on retinopathy pathogenesis are expected because cerebellar stimulation produces a wide range of positive effects on different brain pathologies. *Methods:* The experimental part of the investigation used male Wistar rats with STZ-induced (60.0 mg/kg, i.p.) diabetes. High-frequency (100 Hz) ES was delivered to the VI lobula of the paleocerebellum using two different regimes, with one ES session every two days or thrice ES sessions daily. VEPs were recorded 6 and 12 weeks after diabetes induction. The control groups comprised intact sham-stimulated diabetic rats. VEPs were recorded in patients with newly diagnosed diabetes mellitus after low-intention repeated transcranial magnetic stimulation (rTMS), followed by measurements after sham-rTMS and intensive rTMS. *Results:* The latencies of P1, N1, and P2 increased from 18.8% to 22.3% six weeks after STZ-diabetes induction compared to those of control rats. Chronic high-frequency cerebellar ES prevented the elongation of latency in diabetic rats. This preventive effect of ES was pronounced in rats with intensive ES, and it was not followed by body weight or glucose level modifications. Twelve weeks of ES failed to prevent the enlargement of VEP latency. The P100 latency in patients with diabetes mellitus exceeded those of age-matched controls by 9.6% - 13.5% ($P<0.05$). Photostress after sham stimulation increased the mean VEP latency during the first 20 s, and it did not return to baseline until 60 s of observation. rTMS (1Hz) prevented photostress-induced elongation of the P100 latency, and the mean latency during the post-stress period was not significantly different from that of the control group. *Conclusion:* High-frequency ES of the VI lobula of the paleocerebellar cortex in STZ-induced diabetic rats and cerebellar rTMS in patients with newly diagnosed diabetes mellitus improved the diabetes-induced elongation of VEP wave latency.

Chapter 6 - High cognitive abilities were commonly related to the prefrontal cortex. However, in recent years, the cerebellum was found to be strongly associated with age-related decline in motor and executive functions, even beyond the prefrontal cortex. Theoretical frameworks were suggested to understand the role of the cerebellum: as important for the formation of internal models of behaviour, as important for the timing of behaviour, or as crucial in sequence processing. Imaging research support the idea that age-related changes in cerebellar activation lead to slowed updating of stimulus-response mapping. Here, a meta-analysis of recent findings of cerebellar involvement in executive functions is provided. Also, a methodological issue is raised, relevant for models explaining cerebellar connectivity and effects on cognitive performance in old age. The surprising role of the cerebellum, hence, should no longer be surprising, and research of cognitive decline in old adults should take it under consideration.

In: Development of the Cerebellum
Editor: Severina Fabbri
ISBN: 978-1-53614-317-1

Chapter 1

TIMETABLES OF NEUROGENESIS IN THE DEVELOPMENT OF THE CEREBELLUM

Lucía Rodríguez-Vázquez and Joaquín Martí-Clúa*
Unidad de Citología e Histología, Departamento de Biología Celular, de Fisiología y de Immunología, Facultad de Biociencias, Universidad Autónoma de Barcelona, Bellaterra, Barcelona, Spain

ABSTRACT

The cerebellum is a region of the vertebrate nervous system involved in functions such as motor coordination, perception, cognition and development of the language. The anatomical structure of the adult cerebellum consists of a three-layered cortex and a set of cerebellar nuclei embedded in the white matter. There is evidence indicating that the germinal source of cerebellar neurons is heterogeneous. GABAergic neurons, such as inhibitory interneurons and some deep neurons, originate from the cerebellar neuroepithelium. On the other hand, glutamatergic neurons, including deep cerebellar nuclei neurons and unipolar brush cells, arise from progenitors located in the anterior rhombic lip. Granule cell precursors also originate from the rhombic lip and migrate tangentially over the surface of the cerebellar anlage to form the external granular layer.

* Corresponding Author Email: joaquim.marti.clua@uab.es.

As indicators of DNA synthesis, tritiated thymidine and 5-bromo-2´-deoxyuridine have shown that one of the most important features of the cerebellar development is that each neuronal population is generated during a specific temporal window. This is named timetable of neurogenesis or time of neuron origin. It allows for an accurate delineation of both the onset and cessation of neurogenesis as well as for the determination of the proportion of neurons that are produced during single days of embryonic or postnatal life. We will show here that several types of cerebellar neurons are generated sequentially: first, the output neurons (deep neurons and Purkinje cells) and then, the interneurons (Golgi, unipolar brush, basket, stellate and granule cells).

Keywords: cerebellum; cerebellar cortex; deep cerebellar nuclei; timetable of neurogenesis; neuron

1. Introduction

The cerebellum is an important part of the central nervous system in most vertebrates. This brain structure is involved in several functions, such as motor control, reflex adaptation, motor learning and cognition (Buckner 2013; Lupo et al., 2018). Recent studies have indicated that it also contributes to language and its development (Moberget and Ivry, 2016). The cerebellum is particularly useful in the study of the genesis and the arrangement of neurons, as it has a regular cytoarchitecture formed by two discrete components: the cerebellar cortex in a superficial position and, buried in the cerebellar white matter, an aggregate of neurons that constitutes the deep cerebellar nuclei (DCN). The cerebellar cortex is composed of a limited number of cellular phenotypes that are specifically integrated in the corticonuclear network and that are characterized by distinctive morphologies and molecular markers (Schilling et al., 2008; Chédotal, 2010; Hashimoto and Hibi, 2012). This regular organization has allowed the tracing of the successive stages in the ontogeny of the cerebellar cortex as well as the study of the cellular and molecular mechanisms involved in its development (Altman and Bayer, 1997).

The review will focus on the development of the cerebellum and more specifically on the production of several types of neurons. It will show that these cells are sequentially generated following strict neurogenetic timetables. Taken as a whole, these data indicate that the chronological sequence of neurogenesis throughout the cerebellum is a precisely regulated event. The DCN neurons are the first to be originated. The Purkinje cells (PCs) emerge at some point later than these deep nuclear neurons. The generation of Golgi and unipolar brush cells begins in the prenatal life and continues through the perinatal period. Finally, basket, stellate and granule cells (GCs) are generated in the early postnatal life. We hope these times of neuron origin can be a reference for toxicologists and neurobiologists dealing with developmental abnormalities in the cerebellum.

1.1. Cerebellum Development: An Overview

The adult cerebellar cortex appears to be similarly organized across mammals. This structure is formed by three layers: the molecular layer, whose neuronal components include stellate and basket cells; the Purkinje cell layer, that contains Purkinje and candelabrum cells; and the granule layer, that consists of GCs, Golgi cells, unipolar brush cells and Lugaro cells (Butts et al., 2014; Marzban et al., 2015) (Figure 1).

The immature cerebellum, on the other hand, is composed of four layers. The outermost is the external germinal layer (EGL) formed by small and densely packed cells. This temporary structure produces the most numerous population of cortical neurons: the GCs (Altman and Bayer, 1997) (Figure 2).

In the fetal cerebellar cortex of whales, primates and humans, a fifth layer appears between the Purkinje and inner granular layer. This provisional band is called lamina dissecans (Rakic and Sidman, 1970).

Previous studies have indicated that all cerebellar neurons derive from the most anterior segment of the hindbrain, the rhombomere 1 (Sillitoe and Joyner, 2007; Nakamura et al., 2008).

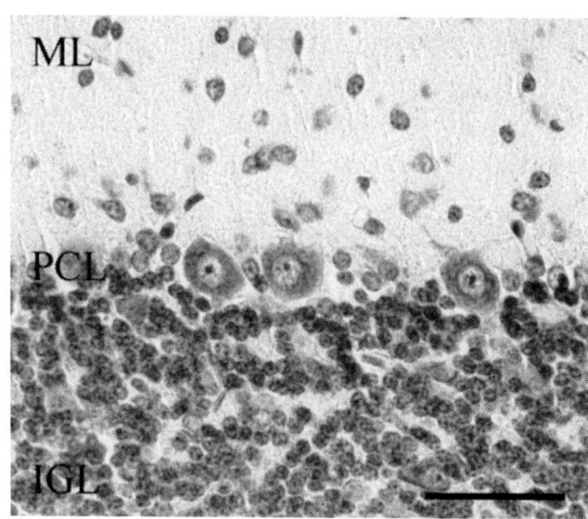

Figure 1. Representative high-magnification photomicrograph of a sagittal section of the vermal cerebellar cortex from a rat collected at postnatal day 90. Stained with toluidine blue. ML: molecular layer; PCL: Purkinje cell layer; IGL: internal granular layer. Scale bar: 30μm.

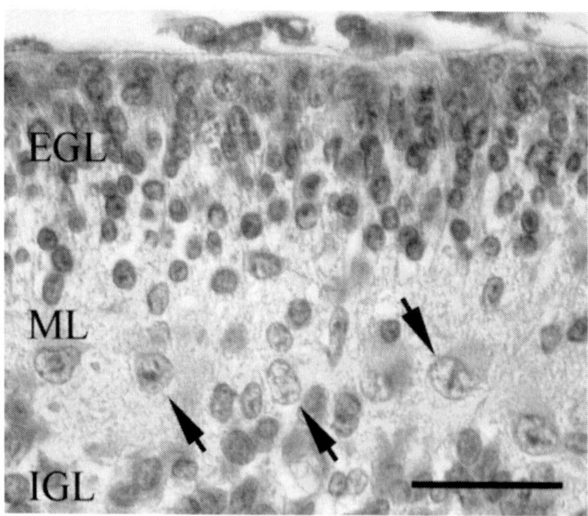

Figure 2. Representative high-magnification photomicrograph of a sagittal section of the vermal cerebellar cortex from a rat injected with 5-bromo-2´-deoxyuridine at postnatal day 9 and killed 2 hours later. The external germinal layer presents a superficial stratum containing the bulk of proliferating cells. 5-bromo-2´-deoxyuridine-postitive cells are those presenting a brown reaction product in their nuclei. EGL: external germinal layer; ML: molecular layer; IGL: internal granular layer. Black arrows indicate Purkinje cells. Scale bar: 30μm.

It has been demonstrated that the isthmic organizer, located at the mesencephalon/rhombomere 1 boundary, directs the formation of cerebellar territory (Yaguchi et al., 2009). In rodents, *Otx2* is expressed in the mesencephalon whereas *Gbx2* is expressed in the metencephalon. These gene expression domains define the mid-hindbrain boundary and allow the formation of the isthmus organizer (Tong et al., 2015).

The organizing activity of the isthmic tissue is mediated by the secreted fibroblast growth factor 8 (Nakamura et al., 2008; Suzuki-Hirano et al., 2010), whose expression is induced by a complex cross-regulatory mechanism involving several transcription factors, such as the LIM homeobox transcription factor 1b (Joiner et al., 2000). Thus, fibroblast growth factor 8 signaling is involved in the survival, specification and patterning of the rhombomere 1 (Yu et al., 2011). After the establishment of the cerebellar territory, neural progenitors emerge from germinal zones and migrate to their final locations within the anlage, where they undergo successive waves of proliferation and migration from the embryonic period until the early postnatal life (Yaguchi et al., 2009).

The establishment of the cerebellar territory is followed by the formation of two germinative compartments with distinct development potentialities: the ventricular neuroepithelium and the anterior rhombic lip. Many lines of evidence have revealed that all cerebellar neurons derive from these areas following regular and precise timetables of neurogenesis. GABAergic neurons, such as PCs, nucleo-olivary neurons, inhibitory interneurons and some deep cerebellar neumostrons, originate from the cerebellar neuroepithelium (Hashimoto and Hibi, 2012). By contrast, glutamatergic neurons, including most deep cerebellar nuclei neurons, unipolar brush cells and projection neurons of the major precerebellar nuclei, arise from progenitors located in the anterior rhombic lip (Leto et al., 2009; 2012; Wullimann et al., 2011). The precursors of GCs also emerge from the rhombic lip, but they migrate tangentially over the pial surface to form a secondary matrix, the EGL (Altman and Bayer, 1997).

1.2. Cerebellar Neurogenesis in the Scenario of Tritiated Thymidine Autoradiography and Bromodeoxyuridine Labeling

The possibility to experimentally identify the proliferating neuron precursors and to follow their fate during the development of the cerebellum began with the application of tritiated thymidine ([^{3}H]TdR) autoradiography in the neuroembryological research (Miale and Sidman, 1961). The technique has generated critical insights into the cellular mechanisms of cerebellum development, including cell kinetics and time of neuron origin (Schultze and Korr, 1981; Altman and Bayer, 1997; Komuro et al., 2001; Martí et al., 2015).

On the other hand, since the introduction of monoclonal antibodies against 5-bromo-2´-deoxyuridine (BrdU) (Graztner 1982), an increasing number of immunocytochemical procedures have been developed for the detection of the BrdU that has been incorporated into replicating DNA (Dolbeare 1995). As compared with [^{3}H]TdR autoradiography, BrdU labeling has provided new advances in the characterization of neuroblast precursors under different experimental contexts concerning the cerebellar development.

Since DNA synthesis can be initiated independently of mitosis, e.g., during gene duplication, repair or apoptosis, [^{3}H]TdR and BrdU are indicators of DNA synthesis and not of cell division (Rakic, 2002; Breunig et al. 2007; Duque and Rakic, 2011).

There are advantages and disadvantages to the use of both markers. Accumulating lines of evidence have revealed that the incorporation of [^{3}H]TdR into cellular DNA induces several harmful dose-dependent effects, including DNA damage and chromosomal aberrations (Ehmann et al., 1975; Kufe et al., 1980; Hu et al., 2002). Moreover, in addition to these effects, [^{3}H]TdR produces changes in cell morphology that are characteristic of cells that have been damaged by ionizing radiation. These alterations included the enlargement of the cell size and the nuclei, and the production of long processes emanating from the cell body (Hu et al., 2002).

Previous studies have indicated that the administration of BrdU to mammalian embryos has teratogenic effects. BrdU alters the development of several regions of the central nervous system (Kolb et al. 1999; Sekerkova et al. 2004a; Kuwagata et al. 2007; Duque and Rakic, 2011) and causes malformations that ultimately lead to behavioral changes (Packard et al., 1974; Bannigan et al., 1990; Shah et al., 1991). In addition to that, BrdU has detrimental effects on the survival of neuroblasts and cell cycle differentiation (Lehner et al., 2011), and it induces senescence in neural progenitors (Ross et al. 2008). Previous data have also indicated that the administration of this halopyrimidine to pregnant dams alters the generative behavior of neuroblasts and promotes their loss during the early development of the cerebellum (Martí et al., 2015; Rodríguez-Vázquez and Martí, 2017).

The detrimental effects of BrdU administration are more severe than those of [^{3}H]TdR (Duke and Rakic, 2011; 2015). This is due to the fact that incorporation of BrdU into replicating DNA produces the faulty base pairing of the bromouracil with guanine instead of adenine. This substitution is related to mutations and breaks in double-stranded DNA that lead to deleterious effects on cell fate and function (Taupin, 2007; Duke and Rakic, 2011; Rowell and Ragsdale, 2012). On the other hand, the only difference between [^{3}H]TdR and the normal endogenous thymidine is an extra neutron in a H atom. Consequently, the structure of the DNA with [^{3}H]TdR is more similar to the DNA of a non-injected animal than the DNA with BrdU (Duke and Rakic, 2011). However, the use of BrdU has become predominant despite its adverse effects.

2. Experimental Design and Histological Procedures

To completely quantify the time course of neuron origin in the cerebellum, both prenatal and postnatal developmental series were used. The animals used in the prenatal series were the offspring of timed-pregnant rats or mice administered with [^{3}H]TdR (New England Nuclear #NET-027) or BrdU (Sigma, St Louis, MO, USA). A group of pregnant dams were injected subcutaneously on two consecutive days with [^{3}H]TdR (5μCi/g of body weight, New England Nuclear no. NET-027) (Bayer and Altman, 1987; Martí et al. 2015). The other pregnant females were administered with six intraperitoneal injections of 6 mg BrdU (Sigma, St Louis, MO, USA, 10mg/ml in sterile saline with 0.007N sodium hydroxide) 8h apart (Sekerkova et al. 2004a; b). Both markers were delivered following the progressively delayed labeling comprehensive procedure (Bayer and Altman, 1987). This method consisted of injecting pregnant dams in an overlapping series in accordance with the following time-windows: embryonic day (E)11-12, E12-13, E13-14, …… E20-E21. The day of sperm positivity was E1. After [^{3}H]TdR or BrdU administrations, the dams gave birth normally.

In the postnatal developmental series, pups were injected with [^{3}H]TdR (5μCi/g of body weight). The injections were progressively delayed between groups (P0+P3, P4+P7, P8+P11,…). The day of birth was P0. All animals were maintained under standard laboratory conditions.

At appropriate times, animals were anesthetized with a ketamine-xylazine mixture (90:10 mg/ml; 1 ml/kg, intraperitoneal) and transcardially perfused with 4% paraformaldehyde in 0.1M phosphate buffer, pH 7.4. Brains were removed from the skulls, weighted, dissected on ice, rinsed in cold PBS and immersed for 36h in the same fixative at 4ºC. Paraffin embedding was carried out following the regular procedures from our laboratory. Serial cerebellar sections (10 μm) were cut in the sagittal plane using a rotary microtome.

2.1. [^{3}H]TDR Autoradiography

Isotope incorporation was detected as previously described (Martí et al. 2002). This consisted of coating the slides with a liquid photographic emulsion (undiluted Kodak NTB3), drying them slowly in a humidified atmosphere and refrigerating them for an exposure time of 12 weeks. The autoradiograms were developed in Kodak D-19. They were lightly post-stained with haematoxylin, dehydrated, and cover-slipped with Permount.

2.2. BRDU Immunocytochemistry

Immunoperoxidase staining for BrdU was performed according to previously published procedure (Molina et al., 2017). Sections were deparaffinized in xylene and rehydrated through a series of graded ethanols. Partial denaturation of DNA was carried out by 3N HCl at 40°C during 15min. Endogenous peroxidase activity was blocked by 3% H_2O_2 for 15 min. Afterwards, slides were washed in 0.5% triton X-100 in PBS, and incubated with a primary antibody (Sigma, clone BU33, Cat. B2531). This antibody was diluted 1:150 in PBS supplemented with 1% bovine sero-albumine (BSA, Boheringer Mannheim, Germany). Following overnight incubation with the primary antibody, sections were incubated with a biotin conjugated goat anti-mouse IgG antibody (Dako) 1:20 for 30 min and then exposed to ExtrAvidin-peroxidase (Sigma) 1:20 for 30 min. Peroxidase activity was developed by adding 3,3'-diaminobenzidine-H_2O_2 (DAB, Sigma) for 5 min. Sections were counterstained with haematoxylin or Feulgen method.

Control sections were prepared replacing the primary antibody by PBS. These routinely showed no immunolabeling.

2.3. Inferring Timetables of Neurogenesis

The determination of the proportion of cells that arise on a particular day required a modification of the progressively delayed comprehensive labelling procedure described by Bayer and Altman (Bayer and Altman, 1987). This method only distinguishes between labeled and unlabeled neurons, and the entire cell population in a given cerebellar region can be used as a source of data. Examples of DCN neurons and PCs from mice injected with [^{3}H]TdR or BrdU are shown in Figures 3A and 3B, respectively.

The major premise of this procedure is that [^{3}H]TdR or BrdU will be incorporated by those neuroblasts engaged in DNA synthesis during marker supply, but not by postmitotic cerebellar neurons. Within a specific population, a maximal percentage (about 95%) of labeled neurons indicates that most precursors are still proliferating at the time of the onset of [^{3}H]TdR or BrdU supply, and few neurons are being generated Specific neuronal populations in the cerebellum are labelled after two consecutive daily injections at some time during development. If the time of the first [^{3}H]TdR or BrdU injections is progressively delayed 24 hours, injections schedules will follow when the percentage of labelled neurons within a specific population declines, reflecting the changes of precursors into young neurons (Bayer and Altman 1987).

The proportion of neurons that are originated each day is related to the daily decline in the percentage of labelled neurons. For instance, the percentage of PCs generated on day E12 is determined as follows: E12 = (% neurons labelled E12 + E13) – (% neurons labelled E13 + E14). An example of how the neurogenesis was inferred throughout the cerebellum is shown in Table 1 (data and calculations for PCs in the vermis).

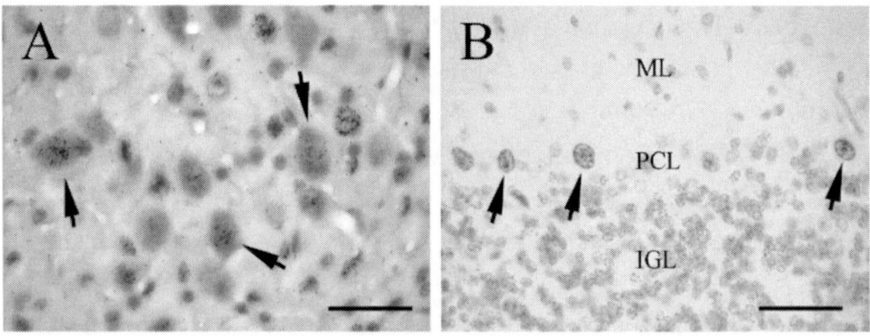

Figure 3. High-magnification photomicrographs of deep cerebellar nuclei neurons (A) and Purkinje cells (B) from mice administered with [^{3}H]TdR (A) or 5-bromo-2´-deoxyuridine (B). Black arrows in A and B show examples of labeled neurons with [^{3}H]TdR and 5-bromo-2´-deoxyuridine, respectively. ML: molecular layer; PCL: Purkinje cell layer; IGL: internal granular layer. Scale bar in A: 30μm. Scale bar in B: 20μm.

Table 1. Neurogenesis of Purkinje cells

Injection group	% labeled neurons	Embryonic day	% Neurons originating
E11-12	95,0 ± 1,5	E10	5,0 ± 0,8%
E12-13	75,2 ± 4,3	E11	19,8 ± 2,1%
E13-14	30,0 ± 6,4	E12	45,2 ± 3,5%
E14-15	3,1 ± 1,2	E13	26,9 ± 2,7%
E15-16	0,0 ± 0,0	E14	3,1 ± 0,4%

Data are represented as means ± SEM of the proportion of Purkinje cells that are labeled with [^{3}H]thymidine and the percentage of Purkinje cells generated. The proportion of generated neurons was inferred by subtracting the proportion of [^{3}H]thymidine-labeled neurons from the proportions of tagged cells of the immediately previous injection series to obtain the proportion of neurons that were produced between the two injections.

3. Development Timetables of the Cerebellar Neurons

The neuronal types that populate the cerebellum are generated following regular and precise timetables of neurogenesis (Altman and Bayer, 1997). These patterns of neuron generation can be altered by internal or environmental factors. To be able to understand these alterations, it is essential to have a previous, detailed knowledge of the cerebellar development. This is possible thanks to the use of ^{3}H]TdR autoradiography and BrdU immunohistochemistry, which allow for the quantitative determination of the birth dates of cerebellar neurons.

In rats, the DCN neurons are the first to be originated. [^{3}H]TdR autoradiography reveals that deep neurons are produced from E13 to E15, with a peak of production on E14 (Altman and Bayer 1997). In mice, on the other hand, patterns of neuron generation show that these neurons are produced from E10 to E13. The peaks of newborn neurons are reached towards E11 (Martí et al., 2001; 2016). (Figure 4 A).

The cerebellar cortex contains several neuronal populations. In rats, autoradiographic studies have shown that PCs are generated somewhat later than DCN neurons. The time of neuron origin profiles reveals that, in the region of the vermis, these macroneurons are generated from E13 to E16, with a peak production on E15 (Altman and Bayer 1997). In mice, the neurogenetic profiles extend from E10 to E14. A substantial number of PCs is produced at E11 (Martí et al., 2001) (Figure 4 A). It is important to highlight that there are systematic differences in the pattern of neurogenesis between mice injected with [^{3}H]TdR and mice injected with BrdU (Martí et al., 2015). These findings have implications for the interpretation of both exogenous markers as indices of cell production.

Rat unipolar brush and Golgi cells are the first interneurons to originate in the cerebellar cortex. The generation of these neurons begins in the prenatal life and continues through the perinatal life (Altman and Bayer 1997; Sekerkova et al., 2004b) (Figure 4 B-C). There are two subgroups of unipolar brush cells. These were defined with the use of antibodies against the ionotropic glutamate receptor GluR2 and calretinin. Their time of neuron origin reveals that an important number of GluR2 and calretinin-positive neurons are originated at E17.5. On the other hand, peaks of newborn neurons GluR2-reactive and calretinin-negative are reached towards E20 (Sekerkova et al., 2004b) (Figure 4 B-C).

Finally, basket cells, stellate neurons and GCs are the last to be originated. In rats, they are produced in the early postnatal life and the times of generation of these neurons overlap. [^{3}H]TdR autoradiography indicates that basket cells have their peak time of origin between P4 and P7, that stellate cells peak between P8 and P11, and that the neurogenesis of the large population of GCs occurs mainly between P8 and P15. No cerebellar neurons are born after P21 (Bayer et al., 1993). (Figure 4 D).

This current review has showed that the generation of cerebellar neurons is sequential. The output neurons (DCN neurons and PCs) are born first and the interneurons (unipolar brush cells, Golgi neurons, basket cells, stellate cells and GCs) last. The cerebellar neurons are produced in overlapping waves to achieve the final cerebellar cytoarchitecture and the organization of the cerebellar circuits. Cortico-nuclear connections (GCs receive inputs from outside of the cerebellum and project to the PCs, the majority of which then project to the DCN neurons) (Butts et al., 2014).

The output from the cerebellum is via the axons of the cerebellar nuclei, most of which travel from the superior cerebellar peduncle to the red nucleus and thalamus. The thalamus, in turn, relays that input to the cerebral cortex (Glickstein and Doron 2008).

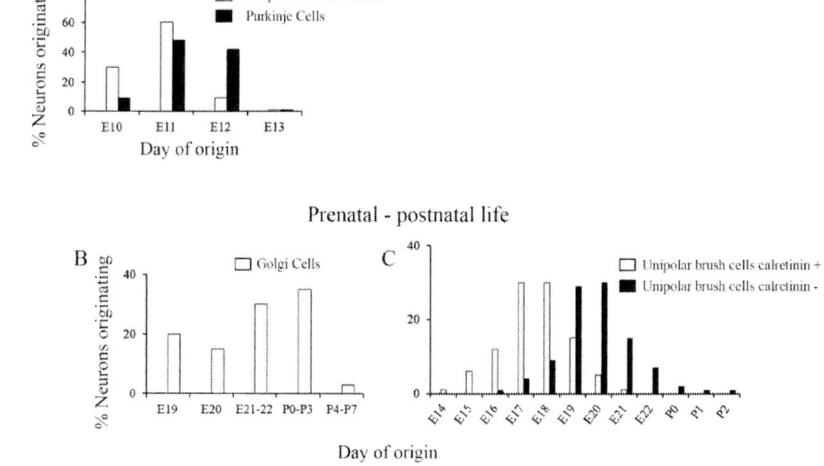

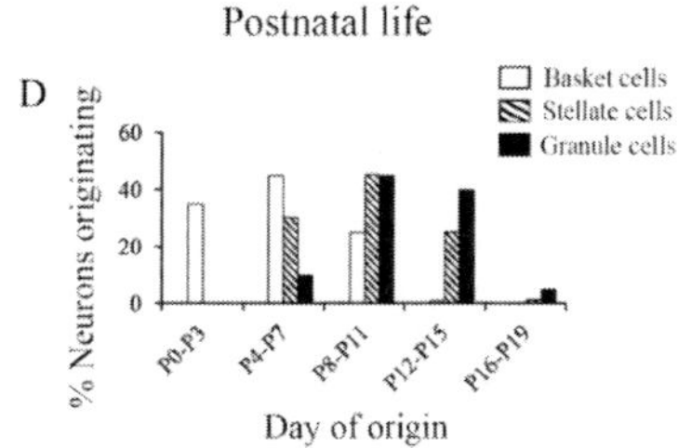

Figure 4. Neurogenesis of cerebellar neurons. Developmental timetables of: (A) deep cerebellar nuclei neurons and Purkinje cells; (B) Golgi cells; (C) unipolar brush cells; (D) basket, stellate and granule cells. The vertical axis indicates the estimated proportion of generated neurons. The horizontal axis indicates the time of generation: prenatal (E10-E22) or postnatal (P0-P19). Modified from Altman and Bayer, 1997 (A, C and D) and Sekerkova et al., (2004).

The alteration of the above-mentioned neurogenetic timetables results in hypoplasia, a permanent reduction of the normal number of neurons. This may produce inappropriate synaptic contacts and affect the cerebellar connectivity. Altered anatomical connections may lead not only to motor impairments, but also to non-motor deficits in complex neurological conditions. In this scenario, cerebellar malfunction is involved in several psychiatric and developmental disorders, including autism spectrum disorders, neuropsychiatric disorders and, intriguingly, type 1 diabetes mellitus (Allin 2016).

REFERENCES

Altman, J., Bayer, S. A. (1997). *Development of the Cerebellar System: In Relation to its Evolution, Structure and Functions.* CRC Press, Inc. Boca Raton.

Allin, M. P. (2016). Novel insights from quantitative imaging of the developing cerebellum. *Semin Fetal Neonatal Med*, 21: 333-338.

Bannigan, J. G. (1985). The effects of 5-bromodeoxyuridine on fusion of the cranial neural folds in the mouse embryo. *Teratology,* 32: 229-239.

Bayer, S. A., Altman, J. (1987). Directions in neurogenetic gradients and patterns of anatomical connections in the telencephalon. *Progress in Neurobiol*, 29: 57-106.

Bayer, S. A., Altman, J., Russo, R. J., Zhang, X. (1993). Timetables of neurogenesis in the human brain based on experimental determined patterns in the rat. *Neurotoxicol*, 14: 83-144.

Breunig, J. J., Arellano, J. I., Macklis, J. D., Rakic, P. (2007). Everything that glitters isn't gold: a critical review of postnatal neural precursor analysis. *Cell Stem Cell* 1: 612-627.

Buckner, R. L. (2013). The cerebellum and cognitive function: 25 years of insight from anatomy and neuroimaging. *Neuron*, 80: 807-15.

Butts, T., Green, M. J., Wingate, R. J. T. (2014). Development of the cerebellum: simple steps to make a little brain. *Development*, 141: 4031-4041.

Chédotal, A. (2010). Should I stay or should I go? Becoming a granule cell. *Trends Neurosci,* 33: 163-172.

Dolbeare, F. (1995). Bromodeoxyuridine: a diagnostic tool in biology and medicine, Part I. Historical perspectives, histochemical methods and cell kinetics. *Histochem J,* 27: 339-369.

Duque, A., Rakic, P. (2011). Different effects of BrdU and ^{3}H-Thymidine incorporation into DNA on cell proliferation, position and fate. *J Neurosci*, 31: 15205-15217.

Duque, A., Rakic, P. (2015). Identification of proliferating and migration cell by BrdU and other thymidine analogs: benefits and limitations. Chapter 7, 123-139. In: Immunocytochemistry and related techniques (Merighi, A., Lossi, L. eds.) *Neuromethods*, vol. 101. Humana Press.

Ehmann, U. K., Williams, J. R., Nagle, W. A., Brown, J. A., Belli, J. A., Lett, J. T. (1975). Perturbations in cell cycle progression from radioactive DNA precursors. *Nature*, 258: 633–636.

Glickstein, M., Doron, K. (2008). Cerebellum: connections and functions. *Cerebellum,* 7: 589-594.

Gratzner, H. G. (1982). Monoclonal antibody to 5-bromo- and 5-iododeoxyuridine. A new reagent for detection of DNA replication. *Science,* 218: 474-475.

Hashimoto, M., Hibi, M. (2012). Development and evolution of cerebellar neural circuits. *Develop Growth Differ*, 54: 373-389.

Hu, V. W., Black, G. E., Torres-Duarte, A., Abramson, F. P. (2002). 3H-thymidine is a defective tool which to measure rates of DNA synthesis. *FASEB Journal*, 16: 1456-1457.

Joyner, A. L., Liu, A., Millet, S. (2000). Otx2, Gbx2 and Fgf8 interact to position and maintain a mid-hindbrain organizer. *Curr Opin Cell Biol,* 2000 12:736-41.

Kolb, B., Pedersen, B., Ballermann, M., Gibb, R., Whishaw, I. Q. (1999). Embryonic and postnatal injections of bromodeoxyuridine produce age-dependent morphological and behavioral abnormalities. *J Neurosci* 19: 2337-2346.

Komuro, H., Yacubova, E., Yacubova, E., Rakic, P. (2001). Mode and tempo of tangential cell migration in the cerebellar external granular layer. *J Neurosci*, 21: 527-40.

Kufe, D. W., Egan, E. M., Rosowsky, A., Ensminger, W, Frei, E. (1980). Thymidine arrest and synchrony of cellular growth in vivo. *Cancer Treat Rep,* 64: 1307-17.

Kuwagata, M., Ogawa, T., Nagata, T., Shioda, S. (2007). The evaluation of early embryonic neurogenesis after exposure to the genotoxic agent 5-bromo-2'-deoxyuridine in mice. *Neurotoxicol,* 28: 780-789.

Lehner, B., Sandner, B., Marschallinger, J., Lehner, C., Furtner, T., Couillard-Despres, S., Rivera, F. J., Brockhoff, G., Bauer, H. C., Weidner, N., Aigner, L. (2011). *Cell Tissue Res,* 345: 313-328.

Leto, K., Bartolini, A., Yanagawa, Y., Obata, K., Magrassi, L., Schilling, K., Rossi, F. (2009). Laminar fate and phenotype specification of cerebellar GABAergic interneurons. *J Neurosci,* 29: 7079.

Leto, K., Rolando, C., Rossi, F. (2012). The genesis of cerebellar GABAergic neurons: fate potential and specification mechanisms. *Front Neuroanat,* 6: 6.

Lupo, M., Olivito, G., Siciliano L., Masciullo, M., Bozzali M., Molinari M., Leggio M. (2018). Development of a Psychiatric Disorder Linked to Cerebellar Lesions. *Cerebellum,* 19: doi: 10.1007/s12311-018-0926-5.

Martí, J., Wills, K. V., Ghetti, B., Bayer, S. A. (2001). Evidence that the loss of Purkinje cells and deep cerebellar nuclei neurons in homozygous weaver mice is not related to neurogenetic patterns. *Int J Dev Neurosci,* 19: 599-610.

Martí, J., Wills, K. V., Ghetti, B., Bayer, S. A. (2002). A combined immnunohistochemical and autoradiographic method to detect midbrain dopaminergic neurons and determine their time of origin. *Brain Res Protoc,* 9: 197-205.

Martí, J., Santa-Cruz, M. C., Serra, R., Hervás, J. P. (2015). Systematic differences in time of cerebellar-neuron origin derived from bromodeoxyuridine immunoperoxidase staining protocols and tritiated thymidine autoradiographic: a comparative study. *Int J Dev Neurosci,* 47: 216-228.

Martí, J., Santa-Cruz, M. C., Hervás, J. P. (2016). Generation and vulnerability of deep cerebellar nuclei neurons in the weaver condition along the anteroposterior and mediolateral axes. *Int J Dev Neurosci,* 49: 37-45.

Marzban, H., Del Bigio, M. R., Alizadeh, J., Ghavami, S., Zachariah, R. M., Rastegar, M. (2015). Cellular commitment in the developing cerebellum. *Front Cell Neurosci* 12, 8: 450.

Miale, I. L., Sidman, R. L. (1961). An autoradiographic analysis of histogenesis in the mouse cerebellum. *Exp Neurol,* 4: 277-296.

Moberget, T., Ivry, R. B. (2016). Cerebellar contributions to motor control and language comprehension: searching for common computational principles. *Ann N Y Acad Sci*, 1369: 154–171.

Molina, V., Rodríguez-Vázquez, L., Owen, D., Valero, O., Martí, J. (2017). Cell cycle division analysis in the rat external granular layer evaluated by several bromodeoxyuridine immunoperoxidase staining protocols. *Histochem Cell Biol,* 148: 477-488.

Nakamura, H., Sato, T., Suzuki-Hirano, A. (2008). Isthmus organizer for mesencephalon and metencephalon. *Dev Growth Differ,* 50 Suppl 1: S113-S118.

Packard, D. S., Skalko, R. G., Menzies, R. A. (1974). Growth retardation and cell death in mouse embryos following exposure to the teratogen bromodeoxyuridine. *Exp Mol Pathol*. 21: 351-362.

Rakic, P., Sidman, R. L. (1970). Histogenesis of cortical layers in human cerebellum, particularly the lamina dissecans. *J Comp Neurol* 139: 473-500.

Rakic, P. (2002) Adult neurogenesis in mammals: an identity crisis. *J Neurosci* 22: 614-618.

Ross, H. H., Levkoff, L. H., Marshall, G. P., Caldeira, M., Steindler, D. A., Reynolds, B. A., Laywell, E. D. (2008). Bromodeoxyuridine induces senescence in neural stem and progenitor cells. *Stem Cells,* 26: 3218-3227.

Rowell, J. J., Ragsdale, C. W. (2012). BrdU birth dating can produce errors in cell fate specification in chick brain development. *J Histochem Cytochem*. 60: 801-810.

Schilling, K., Oberdick, J., Rossi, F., Baader, S. L. (2008). Besides Purkinje cells and granule neurons: an appraisal of the cell biology of the interneurons of the cerebellar cortex. *Histochem Cell Biol,* 130: 601–615.

Schultze, B., Korr, H. (1981). Cell kinetic studies of different cell types in the developing and adult brain of the rat and the mouse: a review. *Cell Tissue Kinet,* 14: 309-325.

Sekerkova, G., Ilijic, E., Mugnaini, E. (2004a). Bromodeoxyuridine administered during neurogenesis of the projection neurons causes cerebellar defects in rat. *J Comp Neurol*, 470: 221-239.

Sekerkova, G., Ilijic, E., Mugnaini, E. (2004b). Time of origin of unipolar brush cells in the rat cerebellum as observed by prenatal bromodeoxyuridine labeling. *Neuroscience,* 127, 845-858.

Shah, R. M., King, K. O., Feeley, E. J. (1991). Pathogenesis of bromodeoxyuridine-induced cleft palate in hamster. *Am. J. Anat,* 190: 219-230.

Sillitoe, R. V., Joyner, A. L. (2007). Morphology, molecular codes, and circuitry produce the three-dimensional complexity of the cerebellum. *Annu Rev Cell Dev Biol,* 23: 549-577.

Suzuki-Hirano, A., Harada, H., Sato, T., Nakamura, H. (2010). Activation of Ras-ERK pathway by Fgf8 and its downregulation by Sprouty2 for the isthmus organizing activity. *Dev Biol,* 337: 284-293.

Taupin, P. (2007). BrdU immunohistochemistry for studying adult neurogenesis: paradigms, pitfalls, limitations, and validation. *Brain Res Rev,* 53: 198–214.

Tong, K. K., Ma, T. Ch., Kwan, K. M. (2015). BMP/Smad signaling and embryonic cerebellum development: stem cell specification and heterogeneity of anterior rhombic lip. *Develop Grwth Differ*, 57: 121-134.

Wullimann, M. F., Mueller, T., Distel, M., Babaryka, A., Grothe, B., Köster, R. W. (2011). The long adventurous journey of rhombic lip cells in jawed vertebrates: a comparative developmental analysis. *Front Neuroanat,* 21: 5-27.

Yaguchi, Y., Yu, T., Ahmed, M. U., Berry, M., Mason, I., Basson, M. A. (2009). Fibroblast growth factor (FGF) gene expression in the developing cerebellum suggests multiple roles for FGF signaling during cerebellar morphogenesis and development. *Dev Dyn,* 238: 2058-72.

Yu, T., Yaguchi, Y., Echevarria, D., Martinez, S., Basson, M. A. (2011). Sprouty genes prevent excessive FGF signalling in multiple cell types throughout development of the cerebellum. *Development,* 138: 2957-68.

In: Development of the Cerebellum
Editor: Severina Fabbri
ISBN: 978-1-53614-317-1

Chapter 2

THE IMPACTS OF MATERNAL DIABETES IN PREGNANCY ON CEREBELLUM DEVELOPMENT IN OFFSPRING

Javad Hami[1,*], PhD, Akram Sadeghi[1,2], PhD, Saeed Vafaei Nezhad[1,2,3] and Ghasem Ivar[4]

[1]Cellular and Molecular Research Center,
Birjand University of Medical Science, Iran
[2]Department of Anatomical Sciences,
Birjand University of Medical Sciences, Iran
[3]Department of Anatomy, School of Medicine,
Shahid Beheshti University of Medical Sciences, Tehran, Iran
[4]Department of Anatomy, School of Medicine,
Birjand University of Medical Sciences, Birjand, Iran

ABSTRACT

There is increasing evidence that maternal diabetes mellitus during the pregnancy period is associated with a higher risk of neurodevelopmental

[*] Corresponding Author Email: javadhami@gmail.com.

and neurofunctional anomalies including motor dysfunctions, learning deficits, and behavioral problems in offspring. The cerebellum is a part of the brain that has long been recognized as a center of movement balance and motor coordination. Moreover, recent studies in humans and animals have also implicated the cerebellum in cognitive processing, sensory discrimination, attention, and learning and memory. Nevertheless the exact mechanisms by which maternal diabetes in pregnancy influence the development of the cerebellum are unclear and further study will be necessary to define the reason for these abnormalities observed in children born to diabetic women.

Results from previous studies demonstrated that multiple biological alterations occur in pregnancies with diabetes and affect the development of fetal central nervous system (CNS), including in uterus hyperglycemia and hyperinsulinemia, neonatal hypoglycemia, and oxidative stress. Recent researches have clearly established that maternal diabetes disrupts the expression of insulin and insulin-like growth factor-1 receptors in the cerebellum of rat newborn. There is also evidence indicating that diabetes in pregnancy disrupts the synaptogenesis in the developing cerebellum.

Here, we review the manuscripts focusing on the negative impacts of maternal diabetes in pregnancy on the developing cerebellar cortex. Dissecting out the mechanisms responsible for maternal diabetes-related changes in the development of cerebellum is helping to prevent from impaired neurocognitive and neurobehavioral functions in offspring.

Keywords: maternal diabetes, cerebellum, rat neonate

1. Introduction

Diabetes is a chronic metabolic disease in which a person has elevated blood glucose levels, either because the body does not produce enough insulin (diabetes Type 1), or because cells fail to respond to insulin (diabetes Type 2) [1, 2]. diabetes Type 1 is induced by autoimmune destruction of insulin-producing pancreatic β-cells and accounts for approximately 10% of the estimated 346 million diabetes mellitus cases worldwide (WHO, 2011) [3, 4]. The remaining 90% of cases are attributed to diabetes Type 2. A third kind of diabetes, known as gestational diabetes, occurs when a pregnant woman develops high blood-glucose levels typically during the second half of pregnancy due to the hormones of pregnancy. Gestational diabetes can revert to normal following pregnancy, but sometimes precedes the development of diabetes Type 2 [5-7]. Recent data of the National Diabetes Fact Sheet shows that total 25.8 million children and adults in the USA (8.3% of the population) have diabetes [8].

All forms of diabetes increase the risk of long-term complications. Up to 67% of adults with diabetes have high blood pressure [9]. Long-term diabetes causes nerve damage in the heart, which can make a heart attack painless or 'silent,' and affects blood vessel formation in the retina of the eye, leading to visual symptoms and sometimes blindness (diabetic retinopathy) [10-12]. High blood sugar can lead to scarring of kidney tissues that may result in chronic kidney diseases (diabetic nephropathy) [11, 13]. Diabetes also affects the nervous system (diabetic neuropathy), causing numbness, tingling and pain in the feet, and increasing the risk of skin damage because of altered sensation [3, 14]. As diabetes affects every part of the body, it can also have devastating complications to the mother and embryo [15].

1.1. Diabetes in Pregnancy

For more than a century, it has been known that diabetes pregnancy can have severe adverse effects on fetal and neonatal outcomes [16-18]. As early as in the 1940s, it was recognized that women who developed diabetes years after pregnancy had experienced abnormally high fetal and neonatal mortality [19]. By the 1950s the term "gestational diabetes" was applied to what was thought to be a transient condition that affected fetal outcomes adversely, then abated after delivery [20]. In the 1960s, O'Sullivan found that the degree of glucose intolerance during pregnancy was related to the risk of developing diabetes after pregnancy [21]. He proposed criteria for the interpretation of oral glucose tolerance tests (OGTTs) during pregnancy that were fundamentally statistical, establishing cut-off values — approximately 2 standard deviations — for diagnosing glucose intolerance during pregnancy. In the 1980s those cut-off points were adapted to modern methods for measuring glucose and applied to the modern definition of gestational diabetes — glucose intolerance with onset or first recognition during pregnancy. While based on O'Sullivan's values for predicting diabetes after pregnancy, the diagnosis of gestational diabetes mellitus (GDM) also identifies pregnancies at increased risk for perinatal morbidity and long-term obesity and glucose intolerance in offspring [22, 23].

Many studies has been shown, infants born to mothers with diabetes have been at significantly greater risk for spontaneous abortion, stillbirth, congenital malformations, and perinatal morbidity and mortality [24, 25]. Fetal and neonatal mortality rates were as high as 65% before the development of specialized maternal and neonatal care. Over the past three decades, practitioners have sought to improve the outcome of diabetic pregnancies so that the results approach those of nondiabetic pregnancies. Subsequently, advances in maternal and fetal care have improved the outlook of the infant of a diabetic mother (IDM) to the point [26, 27]. At which most pregnant women with diabetes can expect to deliver a healthy child when they have received appropriate prenatal care. Currently, 3% to 10% of pregnancies are complicated by abnormal glycemic control. Of these, 80% are caused by gestational diabetes mellitus as opposed to pregestational diabetes mellitus. This number may rise significantly in the next decade as the current significantly overweight pediatric population heads into their child-bearing years [28, 29].

The IDM is at increased risk for periconceptional, fetal, neonatal, and long-term morbidities. The causes of the fetal and neonatal sequelae of maternal diabetes are likely multifactorial; however, many of the perinatal complications can be traced to the effect of maternal glycemic control on the fetus and can be prevented by appropriate periconceptional and prenatal care [30, 31].

Diabetes mellitus during pregnancy period is one of the most common metabolic complications that can be classified into two categories: pre-gestational or gestational diabetes. This metabolic disorder occurs in 3-5 percent of pregnancies. Nevertheless, the prevalence of diabetes in pregnancy has been reported to range between less than 1 percent to about 14 percent in different societies [32].

1.2. The Effects of Diabetes in Pregnancy on Offspring

Several well-done epidemiologic studies have demonstrated a strong association between maternal glycemic control at the time of conception and during early gestation and the incidence of congenital anomalies. Previous studies demonstrated a fourfold higher rate of congenital anomalies of the brain, heart, kidneys, intestine, and skeleton in IDM [33, 34].

By definition, these structural anomalies occur between the periconceptional period and 2 months' gestation, during organogenesis. More than 50% of these anomalies affect the central nervous or cardiovascular systems [35, 36]. The most common neurologic structural abnormalities are related to failure of neural tube closure, including meningomyelocele, encephalocele, and anencephaly [37-39]. Anomalies of the cardiovascular system include transposition of the great vessels, ventricular septal defects, atrial septal defects, and left-sided obstructive lesions, such as hypoplastic left heart syndrome, aortic stenosis, and coarctation of the aorta [36, 40-42].

Periconceptional hyperglycemia also seems to increase the risk of skeletal anomalies. Anomalies include the caudal regression syndrome, which is almost synonymous with IDM, spinal anomalies, and syringomyelia [43, 44]. Renal anomalies include hydronephrosis, renal agenesis, and cystic kidneys [45, 46]. The most common intestinal anomalies include atresias of the duodenum and rectum, although atretic sections may occur anywhere along the length of the gastrointestinal tract [47, 48].

The overall rate of major congenital anomalies in infants born to diabetic mothers is about 6% to 13%, which is approximately 2-3 times higher than that of the normal condition. However, the prevalence of major structural malformations in the children born to mothers with diabetes are to 10 times greater in comparison to the general population. The frequencies of perinatal mortality are also five-fold higher in women with diabetes compared with normal women [49]. The prevalence of Minor congenital anomalies in infants born to 802 mothers with GDM, 117 mothers with PGDM, and 380 normal mothers were assessed by Hod et al. (1992). They found a range between 19.4% and 20.5% in prevalence of minor congenital anomalies in their infant in all groups studied without any marked difference between groups. In their study, there was no correlation between the type and prevalence of minor congenital anomalies with the severity and the time of onset of the diabetes in mothers. Neither there was any relationship between the type or prevalence of minor congenital anomalies with the type or appearance of major congenital anomalies. Overall, the defects in central nervous system, heart, kidney, and skeletal system are among the commonest congenital malformations in the offspring of diabetic pregnancies [50].

Many studies have been done on the effects of maternal diabetes on the nervous system. An increasing number of evidence clearly showed that children born to diabetic mothers are in increased risk of fetal and neonatal anomalies including CNS abnormalities which results in increased infant mortality and morbidity rates [14, 51, 52].

As yet, the exact mechanisms by which maternal diabetes alters the development of growing fetuses are not completely understood, and no distinct teratogenic mechanism has been identified to clearly explain a reason for this range of congenital anomalies observed in the infants born to diabetic mothers. Many of the developmental effects of diabetic pregnancies on the fetus can be attributed to maternal glucose (metabolic) control. In normal pregnancies, the blood glucose level in women remains within a tight range. Consequently, the blood glucose concentration in the fetus is fairly constant as the glucose in the mother's blood crosses the placenta freely. Nevertheless, in pregnancies complicated by DM, there are great variations in the maternal blood glucose level [53, 54].

1.3. Effects of Maternal Diabetes on Developing CNS

The functional and structural effects of diabetes in pregnancy on the developing CNS have been studied in both human and experimental models. Although, the precise mechanisms that diabetes in pregnancy can affect the development and function of nervous system remain to be defined [55-57].

Neurodevelopmental assessment of the offspring born to diabetic dams has been revealed a wide spectrum of behavioral, neurochemical, cellular, and molecular impairments [58, 59]. Experimental models subjected to streptozotocin - induced type 1 diabetic pregnancies developed significant deficits in cognitive behaviors [60]. Kinney et al. [2003] found that the only female offspring born to diabetic dams showed deficits in long-term memory and learning. These results have suggested that the *in utero* diabetic condition has gender-specific effects on CNS development [61]. In a study by Plagemann et al. (1998), alterations in catecholamines levels in the hypothalamic nuclei of newborns born to diabetic animals were evaluated. They reported an increased hypothalamic dopamine (DA) and norepinephrine (NE) concentrations in the offspring born to diabetic rats at birth. Twenty one day-old pups born to diabetic mothers, NE levels were strikingly increased in the ventromedial hypothalamic nucleus and the lateral hypothalamic area (LHA), while DA levels were significantly elevated in the paraventricular hypothalamic nucleus and the LHA. The authors concluded that there are strikingly differences in hypothalamic catecholaminergic systems during early development in the rat newborns born to diabetic animals [62].

Mammalian neural tube is derived from embryonic ectoderm. During early embryogenesis, a portion of the ectoderm is induced to become a layer of neuroectoderm cells called neural plate. The neural plate then folds, elevates and fuses at the dorsal midline to form the neural tube [63-65]. This process is mediated by a number of signaling molecules and transcription factors [66, 67]. Several studies has been shown that maternal diabetes can increases the risk for abnormality in the developing neural tube, leading to neural tube defects (NTD) [68-70]. Mutations in some of these genes have been shown to cause NTDs [71]. The normal development of neural tube also requires the coordination of several biological processes, including cell proliferation and apoptosis in neuroepithelium, which is composed of neural progenitor cells. During development, neural progenitor cells have to make decisions about their positional identities within the neural tube, decide whether to self-renew or undergo mitotic arrest, and decide whether to become a more specified cell type or to undergo apoptosis. Thus, the formation of neural tube depends on accurate coordination of the proliferation, migration, differentiation and apoptosis of neural progenitor cells [72-74]. Dysregulation in this process is detrimental to the neural tube development. Studies have revealed that NTDs can result from alterations in cell proliferation and cell survival of neuroepithelial cells in the developing neural tube [75, 76]. Spina bifida, which results from failure of fusion in the spinal region of neural tube, is among the most common birth defects observed in infants of diabetic mothers [77]. The mechanism underlying the teratogenic effect of maternal diabetes has not been fully understood, but it is believed that the incidence and severity of maternal diabetes-induced congenital malformations are correlated with the degree of maternal metabolic control [78-80]. A series of experimental studies demonstrate that hyperglycemia impairs cell proliferation and induces apoptosis during embryogenesis [31, 81-83]. It has been shown that high glucose inhibits the proliferation of first-trimester trophoblast cells in vitro; hyperglycemic conditions, either in vivo or in vitro, induce apoptosis in rodent blastocysts, and in the neural tube of mouse embryos. In addition, neural progenitor cells isolated from embryonic mouse spinal cord were exposed to different glucose concentrations in vitro to examine the effects of high glucose on the survival, proliferation and apoptosis of neural progenitor cells [84]. It was hypothesized that hyperglycemic conditions affect the proliferation and apoptosis of neural progenitor cells in the developing spinal cord, which could be the cellular mechanism underlying the pathogenesis of maternal diabetes-induced spina bifida [81, 85].

The prevalence of NTDs in the offspring of diabetic mothers is 3 to 10-fold higher than that of in general population [86]. In earlier studies, the mitochondrial morphological changes has been shown in developing neural tubes subjected to a diabetic environment during the same time period when the NTDs are induced in diabetic pregnancies [87].

Previous investigations also report that maternal diabetes is associated with a higher risk of long-lasting neurological impairment that is manifested as deficits in balance and motor coordination, hyperactivity, impairments in attention and memory, and altered social behavior in offspring [88, 89]. In humans, children from mothers with diabetes during pregnancy period may exhibit abnormalities, which include learning defects, motor difficulties, attention deficit, and also the risk of developing schizophrenia [90-92]. Babiker et al. (2007) indicated a higher prevalence of developmental delay and behavioral problems in children born to diabetic women. In that study, growth motor skills and language delay were the major development areas of concern they could link between maternal diabetes and development. There is also evidence demonstrating a negative relationship between the performances of the children born to diabetic mothers with the severity of maternal hyperglycemia [93].

Rizzo et al. (1991) studied the effect of abnormal antepartum maternal glucose and lipid metabolism on the long-range neurobehavioral development of children. Despite vigilant antepartum and obstetric management of maternal diabetes, they found numerous significant correlations between indices of maternal second- and third trimester lipid and glucose regulation and child intellectual performance up to age 11 years. All such correlations suggested that poorer maternal metabolic regulation correlated with poorer child performance on standard measures of neuropsychological functioning [94].

1.4. Effects of Maternal Diabetes on Expression of Insulin and Insulin Like Growth Factor-1 Receptors in Cerebellum

Recent studies found negative effects of maternal diabetes during pregnancy on the development of cerebellar cortex and also the expression and localization of insulin-like growth factor-1 receptor (IGF-1R) and insulin receptor (InsR), as two regulators of central nervous system (CNS) [78, 95, 96].

Experimental investigations in animals indicate a reduction in the numerical densities of neurons in some portions of fetal CNS, especially in the hippocampus and cerebellum due to diabetes during pregnancy which reflects in lower memory and learning skills and defect in memory storage and recall information [97, 98]. A study by Tehranipour and Khakzad (2008) assessed the effect of Streptozotocin (STZ)-induced maternal diabetes on neuronal density in rat neonate's hippocampus immediately after birth. Their data demonstrated that diabetes in pregnancy can reduce the number of hippocampal neurons, especially in the CA3 area [99]. Some investigations have also been demonstrated that fetal hyperglycemia alters the expression of genes that are involved in the proliferation and differentiation of neural cells, indicating the basis for neurodevelopmental and neurocognitive anomalies observed in infants of diabetic mothers [100, 101]. Moreover Previous studies have reveal that, insulin and insulin-like growth factor-1 have neuroprotective anti-apoptotic effects and down-regulation of expression of insulin-like growth factor and its receptor in diabetes might also be expected to lead to neuronal loss and also show Insulin-like growth factor-I (IGF-I) has a crucial role in the regulation of CNS development and growth [102, 103]. It has been reported that the IGF-I stimulates the proliferation of neuronal progenitor cells, increases the survival of neurons and oligodendrocytes, inhibits neural cell apoptosis, and induces differentiation of neurons, including neuritic outgrowth and synaptogenesis, and of oligodendrocytes [104]. In the previous investigation demonstrated that maternal diabetes has a strikingly influence on the cerebellar volumes and numerical density of the IGF-1R-immunoreactive granular and Purkinje cells in various layers of cerebellar cortex of rat neonates in the postnatal days 0, 7, and 14. Haghir et al. evaluate the effects of diabetes in pregnancy on insulin receptor (InsR) and IGF-1 receptor (IGF-1R) expression at mRNA and protein levels in the developing rat cerebellum at P0, P7, and P14. They reported that diabetes during pregnancy strongly influences the regulation of IGF-1R in the developing cerebellum, as a probable mechanism for the neurodevelopmental and neurobehavioral impairments observed in diabetic mothers' Neonates [105]. An investigation by Hernandez-Fonseca et al. (2009) showed an increased apoptosis in pyramidal neurons of cerebral cortex and cerebellar purkinje cells in STZ-induced diabetic rats [106].

Development, in the cerebellum and hippocampus of neonatal rats as a probable mechanism for the neurodevelopmental and neurobehavioral impairments observed in diabetic mothers' neonates. Other investigation by Hami et al. (2016) also evaluated the effects of maternal diabetes on the developing cerebellum of rats. They estimated cerebellar volume, the thickness and the number of cells in the different layers of the cerebellar cortex. Their results have been shown a significant reduction in the cerebellar volume and the thickness of various developing cerebellar cortex such as external granule layer (EGL), molecular layer (ML), and internal granule layer (IGL) in the offspring born to diabetic animals. They also reported that diabetes in pregnancy disrupts the morphogenesis of developing cerebellar cortex and believed that this dysmorphogenesis may be part of the cascade of events through which maternal diabetes affects motor coordination and social behaviors in offspring [107]. Experimental studies revealed that maternal hyperglycemia can cause a significant reduction in gray matter volume rather than to white matter and reduces the number of neurons in the gray matter of the CNS in their offspring [108]. A study by Khaksar and his colleagues (2010) also indicated the detrimental effects of diabetes during pregnancy period on the thickness of cerebellar cortex in neonatal rats [109]. Overall, there are multiple lines of evidence suggesting that the diabetes in pregnancy can causes neurofunctional and neurostructural anomalies in the offspring by alteration of many developmental events such as neurogenesis, migration, and differentiation [17, 31, 110].

With regards to the importance of synaptogenesis in developing cerebellum, here, we have reviewed the related articles focusing on the effects of maternal diabetes during pregnancy on the expression or localization of SYP in the developing cerebellar cortex of neonatal rats. We believe that the neurodevelopmental and neurofunctional impairments observed in the children born to diabetic mothers may be mediated, at least in part, via alterations in expression and localization of SYP in the developing cerebellum [111, 112].

2. Cerebellum

The cerebellum is one of the most studied parts of the brain located at the back of the brain, underlying the temporal and occipital lobes of the brain. For a long time, the cerebellum has been considered to be a critical brain structure for the coordination and control of voluntary movements [113, 114]. However, recent evidence indicates that the cerebellum also plays a role in cognitive, behavioral and emotional functions [115-122]. Several lines of studies clearly indicated that the cerebellum may be involved in a variety of non-motor functions, including sensory discrimination, working memory, semantic association, attention, and verbal learning and memory. Anyway, arranged three-layered cerebellar cortex and well-defined afferent and efferent fiber connections make it a favorite field for research on development and fiber connections of the CNS [123-127].

The cerebellum in rats develops over a long period of time, extending from the early embryonic period until the first postnatal weeks [128, 129]. This protracted development makes it vulnerable to a broad spectrum of developmental abnormalities. The development of the cerebellum occurs in four basic steps: 1) characterization of the cerebellar territory at the boundary between midbrain and hindbrain; 2) formation of two compartments for cell proliferation including the Purkinje cells which arise from the ventricular zone of the metencephalic alar plate and granule cell precursors which formed from the upper rhombic lip; 3) migration of the granule cells: granule precursor cells form the external granular layer (EGL), from which granule cells migrate inwards to their definite position in the internal granular layer (IGL), and 4) formation of cerebellar circuitry and further differentiation. This phenomenon in the developing rat cerebellar cortex has been studied in detail by Altman and colleagues [125-127]. Immediately after birth, granule cells are observed to be aligned outside of the developing cerebellum, known as EGL. At the next postnatal days, the granule cells extrude processes that move towards Purkinje cells. Finally, the cell bodies of the granule cells pass through the layer of Purkinje cells to form IGL. At the same time, Purkinje cells also develop dendrites, and begin to form synapses with parallel fibers, and form the molecular layer (ML). Approximately two weeks after birth, formation of the ML is completed, and the cerebellum shows almost the same morphology as that of the adult rat [95, 105, 130-132].

3. Synapse and Synaptogenesis

Synapses are specialized connections between neurons permitting the controlled transfer of chemical/electrical signals between presynaptic neuronal cells and postsynaptic target neurons. Adequate synapse function is an essential prerequisite of all neuronal processing. True connection between neurons is fundamental to the physiological function of the nervous system, and perception, learning, and memory are only possible when the nervous system is functioning normally [133, 134].

During the development of CNS, synaptogenesis- formation and maturation of synaptic contacts- is one of the most crucial events that is represents the final step of neuronal differentiation. Synaptogenesis begins early in the embryo and extends well into postnatal life. In mammals, the period and length of newly synapse formation is vary widely from species to species which is in human neocortex occurs during the third trimester of gestation and during the first 2 postnatal years, whereas in rodents, the first two weeks after birth represent the most active phase of synaptogenesis. Moreover, formation of a functional synapse is a complex process that involves multiple stages such as axon guidance, synapse formation, synapse maintenance (stabilization), and activity-dependent synapse elimination [135, 136].

Synapses are defined as electrical or chemical depending upon whether transmission occurs via direct propagation of the electrical stimulus in the presynaptic process or via a chemical intermediate. Electrical synapses are gap junctions between neurons and have all the typical structural features of such junctions. They commonly allow bidirectional propagation of the signal, and they play a role in synchronizing neuronal activity. At chemical synapses the presynaptic electrical signal is converted into a secretory response, leading to the release of a chemical intermediate into the synaptic cleft. This chemical message is then reconverted postsynaptically into an electrical signal. Thus chemical synapses are fundamentally asymmetric, although some retrograde, feedback signaling does occur [111, 137-139].

The basic feature of a synapse is a close apposition of specialized regions of the plasma membranes of the two participating cells to form the synaptic interface. On the presynaptic side a cluster of neurotransmitter-filled synaptic vesicles is associated with the presynaptic plasma membrane.

On the postsynaptic membrane an accumulation of neurotransmitter receptors is marked by a thickening of the membrane and by the presence of a submembranous electron dense scaffold.

As soon as they were discovered in the early days of electron microscopy, synaptic vesicles were linked to chemical transmission. They have served ever since as one of the morphological hallmarks of chemical synapses. Synaptic vesicles are small electron-lucent vesicles with a size range of 35-50 nm that store nonpeptide neurotransmitters, such as acetylcholine, glutamate, GABA, and glycine. Within a given nerve terminal they are usually of uniform size, although their diameter and shape may vary slightly in different classes of synapses [133, 137, 140].

The presynaptic cluster can consist of a few dozen to several hundred vesicles at most synapses in the CNS, but it may contain up to thousands of vesicles at specialized synapses. In some very large terminals (such as those of the mossy fiber endings in the hippocampus and cerebellum) a single large cluster of synaptic vesicles is connected to multiple, independent synaptic junctions with distinct postsynaptic elements [141, 142].

The cluster of vesicles is very compact at some synapses and more dispersed at others. Interactions underlying vesicle clustering may vary with the distance from the presynaptic membrane. At each synapse a few vesicles are in physical contact with the presynaptic plasma membrane at release sites ("docked vesicles"), also called "active zones" [139, 143].

Synapses display a wide range of properties. Some cells are connected by a single synaptic contact site, whereas others are connected by many, and the number of active zones per contact varies from one to hundreds. At some synapses a presynaptic action potential reliably triggers vesicle fusion at a single synaptic contact, whereas at others an action potential rarely triggers vesicle fusion.

A key feature of neurotransmitter release is that it involves fusion of the membrane of synaptic vesicles with the presynaptic plasma membrane, a process that is tightly regulated by calcium. After exocytosis, vesicles are endocytosed and recycled. As a result, synaptic vesicles undergo a cycle of membrane traffic composed of exocytosis, endocytosis, and recycling [144, 145].

Chemical synapses are best characterized as asymmetric neuronal junctions which are composed of three compartments: the presynaptic bouton, the synaptic cleft and the postsynaptic apparatus. Presynaptic boutons generally form along the long axis of axons and are filled with anywhere from neurotransmitter substances filled synaptic vesicles such as glutamate, acetylcholine, glycine, dopamine, serotonin, adrenalin, noradrenalin or gamma amino butyric acid (GABA). These vesicles are often released in an activity dependent manner into the small space between the pre-and post-synaptic membranes also called synaptic cleft. In the synaptic cleft, they bind and activate neurotransmitter receptors within the postsynaptic membrane. In fact, the most principal function in the presynaptic buttons is the regulated release of neurotransmitter in a tightly regulated process called exocytosis which is accomplished through the fusions of synaptic vesicles with the presynaptic membrane [142, 146-149].

3.1. The Synaptic Vesicle Cycle

The synaptic vesicle cycle can be envisioned to start with the uptake of neurotransmitters into synaptic vesicles via ATP driven transport. Uptake is mediated by specific transport proteins that are specialized for the various transmitters. Synaptic vesicles filled with neurotransmitter move to the active zone of the presynaptic plasma membrane in a translocation process which is most likely mediated via a molecular motor. At the active zone, the vesicles become attached or "docked" to the plasma membrane [150-152].

Docking involves the specific interaction between the vesicles and the active zone; the vesicles do not seem to attach to any other part of the presynaptic plasma membrane. Calcium then triggers the completion of fusion in a rapid reaction that can occur in less than 0.1 ms. Fusion can occur via two mechanisms. The first involves the complete uptake of the vesicle into the presynaptic plasma membrane (full fusion), and the second involves the opening of a transient fusion pore which allows neurotransmitter release but also allows the vesicle to retain its identity as a vesicle and be quickly retrieved back into the vesicle pool without having to go through full fusion (kiss-and-run) [153-155].

After exocytosis vesicular proteins are recycled back into synaptic vesicles via clathrin-mediated endocytosis which occurs away from the active zone on the periphery of the synaptic bouton. Vesicle transport, target recognition, docking, and fusion each involve the ordered and sequential recruitment of protein complexes from the cytoplasm. The membrane constituents of the organelle are ultimately responsible for orchestrating association of the complex, task execution, and complex disassembly. Recent work has shown that the synaptic vesicle proteome is quite extensive [156-158].

The major proteins which are involved in the aforementioned vesicle recycling process are: Synaptotagmin (Syt) which is thought to be the main calcium sensing protein on the synaptic vesicle surface, Synaptobrevin (Syb) or the V-SNARE also found on the vesicle surface, and Syntaxin (Syx) or the T-SNARE found on the presynaptic membrane. These three proteins, along with Soluble-NSF-Attachment- Protein-25 (SNAP-25) make up the SNARE complex which is thought to be the main facilitator of calcium mediated synaptic vesicle fusion [142, 159, 160].

Neurotransmitter release is a highly regulated process comprised of a series of steps that include: the targeting of SVs to pre-synaptic active zones, the anchoring of SVs to the plasma membrane, the fusion of the SV membrane with the plasma membrane upon stimulation, and the recycling of the SV membrane and machinery back into a functional SV [161].

Synaptic transmission starts with the arrival of an action potential at a pre-synaptic terminal (bouton). The action potential results in depolarization of the membrane potential in the presynaptic terminal and triggers opening of voltage-gated calcium channels. Extracellular Ca2+ ions flow into the intracellular compartment through the calcium channels [162].

SV proteins play a crucial role in determining spatiotemporal profile of major neurotransmitters in the CNS. There are a large number of pathological conditions that are associated with abnormal neuro-transmission. Treatment of these conditions, therefore, relies heavily upon better understanding of the SV cycle. SV membrane proteins play a major role in regulating the SV cycle and the neurotransmitter release, thus are emerging as promising targets for drugs of important neuropathological conditions [160, 163].

For example, a recent genetic study has established a direct correlation between synaptophysin and a cognitive deficit, suggesting that this protein could be an important target for enhancing cognitive functions. Defects in SV cycle are commonly found prior to neuronal losses in Parkinson's disease and Alzheimer's disease [164-166]. In summary, this study will shed light on the general understanding of synaptic function and development of treatments for pathological conditions of the CNS [167].

If a sufficient number of Ca2+ ions bind to the Ca2+ sensor protein on SVs, this binding triggers activation of effector proteins which mediate fusion between synaptic vesicles (SVs) and the presynaptic plasma membrane. Neurotransmitter is then released from SVs and binds to postsynaptic receptors, which results in depolarization or hyperpolarization of the postsynaptic neuron [168, 169].

Several lines of studies were carried out to characterize the components of the synaptic vesicle membrane and found a number of proteins, including synaptophysin, synaptogamin and etc. that functions as the regulators of exocytosis [142, 159-161].

3.2. Synaptophysin

Syp1 is a member of the physin family which consists of synaptophysin, synaptoporin, pantophysin (sypl1), mitsugumin (sypl2), and synaptogyrin. Physiologically it has been observed that Syp1 undergoes a major cellular redistribution in schizophrenia, although how this relates to the disease is unclear. Syp1 is a 38 kDa integral membrane protein which is a member of the MARVEL (MAL and Related proteins for VEsicle trafficking and membrane Link) family of integral membrane proteins associated with membrane juxtapositions [170, 171].

Despite being the most abundant synaptic vesicle membrane protein, the function of synaptophysin remains enigmatic. For example, synaptic transmission was reported to be completely normal in synaptophysin knockout mice; however, direct experiments to monitor the synaptic vesicle cycle have not been carried out. Here, using optical imaging and electrophysiological experiments, we demonstrate that synaptophysin is required for kinetically efficient endocytosis of synaptic vesicles in cultured hippocampal neurons. Truncation analysis revealed that distinct structural elements of synaptophys in differentially regulate vesicle retrieval during and after stimulation. Thus, synaptophysin regulates at least two phases of endocytosis to ensure vesicle availability during and after sustained neuronal activity [172-174].

Synaptophysin (syp) was the first synaptic vesicle (SV) protein to be cloned and characterized, and is now known to belong to a family of proteins with four transmembrane domains that includes synaptogyrin (syg) and synaptoporin. Syp is the most abundant SV protein by mass, accounting for ~10% of total vesicle protein. Each SV harbors ~32 copies of syp, which is second only to synaptobrevin (8% of the total SV protein) at ~70 copies per vesicle. Because syp is exclusively localized to SVs, it is widely used as a marker for pre-synaptic terminals [175-177].

Structurally, syp spans the vesicle membrane four times with a short amino- and a long carboxyterminal tail, both of which are exposed on the cytoplasmic surface of the SV membrane. In addition, there are two short intravesicular loops that contain disulfide bonds. Syp is N-glycosylated on the first intravesicular loop and is phosphorylated on the long cytoplasmic tail; the function of these posttranslational modifications remain unknown. Based on amino acid sequences the predicted secondary structure of mammalian Syp consists of four transmembrane α-helices, two intravesicular loops, and cytoplasmic N- and C-termini. The C-terminus contains a Ca2+ binding motif and ten pentapeptide repeats, nine of which contain tyrosine residues which are phosphorylated by Src*in vitro* [178-180].

There is evidence suggesting that syp, especially its four transmembrane domains, may promote formation of highly curved membranes as in small

SVs. Indeed, ectopic expression of syp alone in non-neuronal cells leads to formation of small cytoplasmic vesicles. A recent electron microscopy study revealed that syp forms hexameric structures that are similar to connexons [160, 181-183].

Previous molecular studies have hinted at a number of diverse roles for syp in synaptic function including exocytosis, synapse formation, biogenesis and endocytosis of SVs. Surprisingly, mice lacking syp were viable and had no overt phenotype [176, 184]. Synaptic transmission, and the morphology or shape of SVs, were not altered in syp knockout mice. Recent genetic screening in human subjects, and behavioral studies in mice, have implicated loss or truncation of syp in mental retardation and/or learning deficits. These new results suggest that syp might play a subtle yet important role in regulating synaptic transmission in neuronal circuits involved in learning and memory. Synaptophysin mRNA is expressed early in development, and synaptophysin protein levels increase significantly during periods of synapse formation.

Therefore, it is suggested that SYP is involved in calcium dependent synaptic vesicle exocytosis. In the previous investigations, SYP has also been considered as a reliable marker for synaptic density and synaptogenesis [180, 181, 185, 186].

The expression of SYP already starts during early neurogenesis in embryonic developing brain and is greatly up-regulated during synaptogenesis. There is also evidence demonstrating that upregulation of SYP expression may contribute to the mechanisms underlying learning and memory. Conversely, aberrant SYP expression has been associated with several psychiatric disorders and neurodegenerative diseases, such as, Parkinson disease, and Alzheimer's disease. Earlier studies on aging and neurodegenerative disorders have correlated change in SYP immunoreactivity with loss or increase in synaptic densities [187-190]. In a study by Thome et al. (2001), the researchers revealed that stress exposure leads to the reduction in hippocampal expression of SYP [191].

3.3. Effects of Maternal Diabetes in Pregnancy on Synaptogenesis in Developing Cerebellum

The adverse impacts of diabetes during pregnancy period on the developing CNS of the fetuses and newborns are already well documented [31, 82, 83, 88, 90, 107]. However, there is limited number of studies that specially focused on the impacts of diabetes during pregnancy period on synaptogenesis in the developing cerebellum of offspring.

Both PGDM and GDM can affect fetal neurodevelopment. Although the untoward effects of maternal diabetes on pregnancy outcomes with respect to congenital malformations have generally been appreciated, the effect of maternal diabetes on the development of central nervous system (CNS) in the fetuses and its behavioral sequelae remains to be completely defined. A limited number of long-term follow-up studies of neurodevelopmental outcomes in diabetic pregnancies have been reported [84, 192, 193]. Nevertheless, it is demonstrated that children born to diabetic mothers are more likely to have neurodevelopmental abnormalities including impairments in learning ability, activity level, attention span, and motor functioning [89, 110]. Interestingly, some of these deficiencies are well-known as risk factors in children who develop schizophrenia later, but the degree of risk is variable and may be related to the severity of metabolic derangement in the mothers with diabetes [194]. Examination of cognitive functioning and the behavior of the children born to diabetic mothers offer the opportunity to functionally assess the CNS development. Hence the assessment of the behavior and cognition in the offspring of diabetic mothers may clarify the maternal diabetes effects on the development of CNS. The results of earlier studies clearly demonstrated that the diabetes during pregnancies may results in intellectual and behavioral functioning disturbances in the infants. These data suggest a teratogenic effect of diabetes in pregnancy on the function of CNS in fetuses and provides the earliest indicator of postnatal CNS deficiencies reflected in intellectual and behavioral problems observed in the children of mothers with diabetes and also Earlier reports on the neurologic development in infants of diabetic mothers revealed serious CNS deficits, even in the absence of structural malformations. These alterations were significantly less severe when maternal diabetes was medically controlled and treated, but some alterations in cognitive function may persist throughout childhood [78, 92, 195].

When pregestational and gestational diabetes-exposed children were grouped together in the study of DeBoer et al. (2005), it was demonstrated a negative link between maternal diabetes and development of memory, circuitry, and behavioral mnemonic performance in children at 1-year of age. Moreover, they showed that the metabolic abnormalities due to diabetes during pregnancy alters prenatal development, which can influence memory performance on a delay recall task [196].

The earlier investigations demonstrated a moderate disturbance in memory and learning and complex information processing of offspring born to mothers who had diabetes during their pregnancy. Rizzo and colleagues (1991), in their investigation demonstrated a significant correlation between gestational diabetes and lower IQ in children [94].

Interestingly, Xiang et al. (2015) found a close relationship between intrauterine exposures to preexisting or gestational diabetes mellitus (GDM) with increased risk of autism spectrum disorder (ASD) in the offspring [197].

Other studies also revealed a negative relationship between the severity of maternal hyperglycemia during and the gestation and the performance of the children on various developmental and behavioral tests. A research by Ornoy et al. (2001) reported that children younger than 9 years, born to diabetic women, had a higher rate of attention deficit, lower cognitive scores, and lower gross and fine motor achievements [92]. In another study, Rizzo et al. (1991) revealed a striking relationship between second- and third-trimester glycemic control and poorer infant responses on the Brazelton Neonatal Behavioral Assessment Scale [198]. Taken together, the existing evidence not only demonstrate the teratogenic effect of maternal diabetes on the development of offspring's nervous system, but also provide the perhaps earliest indicator of postnatal CNS problems reflected in intellectual, behavioral and movement anomalies exhibited by children of mothers with diabetes. Nevertheless, no report can fully explore the molecular mechanisms of maternal diabetes-induced neurodevelopmental and neurofunctional abnormalities.

In a recent study by Hami et al., (2016), the authors evaluated the effects of diabetes in pregnancy on the expression and localization of SYP during the development of cerebellum in the rat offspring. The authors found no significant alterations in the cerebellar expression/localization of SYP in neonate's born to diabetic animals, immediately after birth. Nevertheless, they reported that the expression of SYP was significantly down-regulated at one- and two- weeks old of age rats. In addition, their results also demonstrated that the localization of SYP protein was strikingly reduced in all three distinct layers of cerebellar cortex of neonates born to diabetic animals, especially at postnatal day (P) 14 [111]. Another recent study by Vafaei-Nezhad et al. (2016) indicated that there were no differences in the SYP expression/localization in the hippocampus of neonates born to diabetic dams at P0; the researchers also indicated that the gestational diabetes in pregnancy is associated with a significant downregulation in hippocampal expression/localization of SYP in the neonatal rats at P7, and P14 [140]. Since SYP and other synaptic vesicle proteins have been implicated in the mechanisms of cellular plasticity underlying learning; the early decrease in SYP expression/localization may reflect a downregulation of synaptic function and may be related to the reduction in synaptic density and might disrupt the development and function of cerebellum.

Taken together, the exact mechanisms through which diabetes in pregnancy affects fetal CNS development and function are not completely understood, the conclusion from review of numerous studies is that maternal hyperglycemia during pregnancy may be a major teratogenic factor. Maternal diabetes mellitus during pregnancy is characterized by glucose intolerance and insulin absence or resistance. Mothers with glucose intolerance are frequently treated with exogenous insulin to maintain normoglycemia. Whereas maternal glucose traverses the human placenta relatively easily, maternally derived or exogenously given insulin does not. The fetus becomes hyperglycemic and stimulates islet cell proliferation and insulin production. As long as maternal glycemic status is controlled and transplacental glucose delivery remains steady, fetal glucose metabolism remains stable. Fetal glucose metabolism is most likely to be compromised by wide swings in maternal serum glucose concentrations caused by inconsistent maternal glycemic control. Periods of chronic maternal (and fetal) hyperglycemia result in accelerated fetal growth, whereas sudden reductions in maternal glucose concentrations place fetuses with islet cell hyperplasia at an increased risk for hypoglycemic episodes. Both events have been implicated in the increased fetal mortality rate seen in diabetic pregnancies [55, 112, 199].

Several lines of studies also emphasized the direct correlation between high blood glucose concentrations in mothers as revealed by increased level of glycosylated hemoglobin (HbA1c) with increased frequency of congenital malformations in offspring. Towner et al. (1995) found a striking correlation between pregestational elevated HbA1c in early pregnancy with the increased risk of fetal congenital malformations. There is enough evidence accumulates to support this hypothesis that the tight glycemic control in early and before pregnancy may reduce the frequency of anomalies in the infants born to diabetic mothers [200]. Therefore, the prevalence of congenital abnormalities in children born to mothers with diabetes has decreased in the last three decades probably as a result of the overall progress in monitoring of blood glucose concentrations in diabetic pregnant women [201, 202].

The remarkable thing about the glucose, in contrast to insulin, is that Glucose can freely cross the placental barrier; thus, maternal hyperglycemia during gestational period causes fetal hyperglycemia. Fetal hyperglycemia stimulates the developing, resulting to *In utero* fetal hyperinsulinemia. On separation of the newborn from the mother, the glucose former no longer is supported by placental glucose transfer, may develop neonatal hypoglycemia [35, 203].

Thereafter, fetal hyperglycemia stimulates the pancreatic b-cell hypertrophy and hyperplasia in the developing fetus resulting in increased insulin secretion and consequently, in utero hyperinsulinemia affects different parts of the developing CNS [204].

Chronic fetal hyperglycemia and hyperinsulinemia affect the fetal basal metabolic rate, with secondary effects on fetal oxygenation and erythropoiesis. Fetal hyperglycemia and fetal hyperinsulinemia increase fetal total body oxygen consumption by as much as 30% in a relatively oxygen-limited environment. Although the fetus increases its rate of substrate uptake and oxidation, the human placenta has limited ability to increase oxygen delivery in the face of increased demand. Oxygen transport may be further complicated by placental vascular disease, particularly in women with more advanced diabetes. The resultant relative fetal hypoxemia likely contributes to the increased incidence of fetal death, metabolic acidosis, erythropoiesis, and alterations in fetal iron distribution. The fetus responds to the relative hypoxemia by increasing oxygen carrying capacity. IDMs have elevated cord serum erythropoietin concentrations that indicate fetal hypoxemia. Primate and sheep models demonstrate that this effect is chronic and results in polycythemia and altered iron distribution. In humans, the severity of polycythemia is directly related to lack of maternal glycemic control [205-208].

Although hyperglycemia is thought to be a major teratogenic factor in diabetic pregnancy; some researchers believe that maternal metabolic condition (e.g., triglycerides and β-hydroxybutyrate levels, and branched chain amino acids) in combination with a disturbed fetal metabolism of sorbitol, inositol, arachidonic acid and prostaglandins could have a teratologic significance and thus be important for the occurrence of fetal abnormalities [209, 210]. An excess of fetal reactive oxygen species (ROS) has also been implicated in the etiology of diabetes-induced congenital malformations. These free radicals contribute to increase neuronal death by oxidizing proteins, damaging DNA, and inducing the lipoperoxidation of cellular membranes. In vitro and in vivo studies have shown that the disturbed development of embryos in a diabetic milieu can be normalized by treatment with different antioxidants including Vitamins C, E, etc. [211-214].

The results of earliest studies clearly demonstrated that the diabetes during pregnancy can effect on iron metabolism. The functional consequences of fetal iron redistribution and organ iron deficiency are being investigated. Iron is an important factor in cell growth and energetics. Early postnatal iron deficiency results in myopathies and altered neurodevelopment. It is plausible that iron deficiency compromises fetal wellbeing, which makes the fetus of the mother with diabetes at higher risk for morbidity and mortality [215-217].

In theory, compromised non-heme tissue iron status (e.g., heart and brain) results in similar myopathy and abnormal neurologic functioning that is seen in infants with postnatal iron deficiency. If this is the case, tissue iron deficiency may provide a partial explanation for the fragility of these infants in the newborn intensive care unit. Iron-deficient infants are at increased risk for neurodevelopmental and neurobehavioral abnormalities. Animal models demonstrate that gestational and early postnatal iron deficiency affects myelination, brain energy metabolism, and brain monoamine neuro-transmitter metabolism. Perinatal iron deficiency seems to increase the vulnerability of the neonatal brain, particularly the hippocampus, to hypoxic-ischemic insult. Perinatal iron deficiency may place IDMs, who have an increased risk of acute and chronic hypoxemia, at even greater risk of perinatal brain injury. A recent study provided evidence that IDMs demonstrate abnormal cognitive processing in the newborn period and that this effect may be related partly to iron status [218-222].

Additionally, some researchers argue that the maternal metabolic condition, in combination with a disturbed fetal metabolism, may have teratogenic consequences and may increase the risk of fetal abnormalities in diabetic pregnancies [223, 224].

Some study also show that The recent reports that the cytokine necrosis factor-alpha (TNF) plays a role in both insulin and noninsulin-dependent gestational diabetes raises additional questions as to the causes of long term neurodevelopmental abnormalities in the IDM [225]. Coughlan et al. studied placental and adipose tissue from normal and gestational diabetic mothers. When these tissues were incubated with exogenous glucose significantly increased amounts of TNF was released from the tissues of diabetic mothers as compared to controls. TNF, which crosses the placenta, has been implicated to be neurotoxic to the developing brain of the fetus and has been correlated with increased incidence and severity of white matter damage and cerebral palsy [226].

Some works has been shown that Ketones in the mother's blood readily cross the placenta, but they cannot be cause fetal hyperinsulinemia; so, they might not influence fetal growth and development [35].

In diabetic pregnancies in rats, it is clearly established that the elevated intracellular free oxygen radicals concentrations have been accompanied by the increased risk of embryopathies [227, 228]. Nevertheless, hyperglycemia-induced fetal malformations in rodents have been demonstrated to associate with the number of genomic DNA mutations [229]. Therefore, there are animal studies showing that the free radical scavengers and antioxidants may decrease the risk of teratogenicity of maternal diabetes.

CONCLUSION

In these studies using SYP, a marker of synaptic density and synaptic vesicle formation, it was shown that maternal hyperglycemia, in combination with neonatal hyperinsulinemia was able to decline synaptogenesis in the offspring's cerebellar cortex. This alteration may result in a delay in normal cerebellar development and function, and could be a reason for the structural, behavioral, and cognitive abnormalities observed in the offspring of diabetic mothers.

REFERENCES

[1] Daneman D. Type 1 diabetes. *The Lancet.* 2006;367(9513):847-58.

[2] Quinn L. Type 2 diabetes: epidemiology, pathophysiology, and diagnosis. *The Nursing Clinics of North America.* 2001;36(2): 175-92, v.

[3] Boulton AJ, Vinik AI, Arezzo JC, Bril V, Feldman EL, Freeman R, et al. Diabetic neuropathies: a statement by the American Diabetes Association. *Diabetes care.* 2005;28(4):956-62.

[4] Whiting DR, Guariguata L, Weil C, Shaw J. IDF diabetes atlas: global estimates of the prevalence of diabetes for 2011 and 2030. *Diabetes research and clinical practice.* 2011;94(3):311-21.

[5] Farrar D, Duley L, Lawlor DA. Different strategies for diagnosing gestational diabetes to improve maternal and infant health. *Cochrane Database Syst Rev.* 2011;10.

[6] Teh WT, Teede HJ, Paul E, Harrison CL, Wallace EM, Allan C. Risk factors for gestational diabetes mellitus: implications for the application of screening guidelines. *Australian and New Zealand Journal of Obstetrics and Gynaecology.* 2011;51(1):26-30.

[7] Mandelbrot L, Legardeur H, Girard G. Screening for gestational diabetes mellitus: Is it time to revise the recommendations? *Gynecologie, obstetrique & fertilite.* 2010;38(6):409-14.

[8] Hunt KJ, Schuller KL. The increasing prevalence of diabetes in pregnancy. *Obstetrics and Gynecology Clinics.* 2007;34(2):173-99.

[9] Devereux RB, Roman MJ, Paranicas M, O'grady MJ, Lee ET, Welty TK, et al. Impact of diabetes on cardiac structure and function: the strong heart study. *Circulation.* 2000;101(19):2271-6.

[10] Malani PN. Harrison's principles of internal medicine. *JAMA.* 2012;308(17):1813-4.

[11] Lefèbvre PJ, Scheen AJ. Management of non-insulin-dependent diabetes mellitus. *Drugs.* 1992;44(3):29-38.

[12] Vidyasari R, Sovani I, Mengko T, Zakaria H, editors. *Vessel enhancement algorithm in digital retinal fundus microaneurysms filter for nonproliferative diabetic retinopathy classification.* Instrumentation, Communications, Information Technology, and Biomedical Engineering (ICICI-BME), 2011 2nd International Conference on; 2011: IEEE.

[13] Kurt M, Atmaca A, Gürlek A. Diyabetik nefropati. *Acta Medica.* 2004;35(1):12-7.

[14] Galer BS, Gianas A, Jensen MP. Painful diabetic polyneuropathy: epidemiology, pain description, and quality of life. *Diabetes research and clinical practice.* 2000;47(2):123-8.

[15] Alberti K, Eckel RH, Grundy SM, Zimmet PZ, Cleeman JI, Donato KA, et al. Harmonizing the metabolic syndrome: a joint interim

statement of the international diabetes federation task force on epidemiology and prevention; national heart, lung, and blood institute; American heart association; world heart federation; international atherosclerosis society; and international association for the study of obesity. *Circulation.* 2009;120(16):1640-5.

[16] Ovesen PG, Jensen DM, Damm P, Rasmussen S, Kesmodel US. Maternal and neonatal outcomes in pregnancies complicated by gestational diabetes. A nation-wide study. *The Journal of Maternal-Fetal & Neonatal Medicine.* 2015;28(14):1720-4.

[17] Sadeghi A, Esfandiary E, Hami J, Khanahmad H, Hejazi Z, Razavi S. Effect of maternal diabetes on gliogensis in neonatal rat hippocampus. *Advanced biomedical research.* 2016;5.

[18] Sweeting AN, Ross GP, Hyett J, Molyneaux L, Constantino M, Harding AJ, et al. Gestational diabetes mellitus in early pregnancy: evidence for poor pregnancy outcomes despite treatment. *Diabetes Care*. 2016;39(1):75-81.

[19] Miller HC, Hurwitz D, Kuder K. Fetal and neonatal mortality in pregnancies complicated by diabetes mellitus. *Journal of the American Medical Association.* 1944;124(5):271-5.

[20] Worcester J, Stevenson SS, Rice RG. 677 Congenitally Malformed Infants and Associated Gestational Characteristics: II. Parental Factors. *Pediatrics.* 1950;6(2):208-22.

[21] Bleicher SJ, O'Sullivan JB, Freinkel N. Carbohydrate metabolism in pregnancy: The interrelations of glucose, insulin and free fatty acids in late pregnancy and post partum. *New England Journal of Medicine.* 1964;271(17):866-72.

[22] Skyler JS, O'Sullivan MJ, Robertson EG, Skyler DL, Holsinger KK, Lasky IA, et al. Blood glucose control during pregnancy. *Diabetes Care.* 1980;3(1):69-76.

[23] O'Sullivan JB. Establishing criteria for gestational diabetes. *Diabetes care.* 1980;3(3):437-9.

[24] Greene MF, Hare JW, Cloherty JP, Benacerraf BR, Soeldner JS. First-trimester hemoglobin A1 and risk for major malformation and spontaneous abortion in diabetic pregnancy. *Teratology.* 1989;39(3): 225-31.

[25] Kitzmiller JL, Buchanan TA, Siri K, Combs AC, Ratner RE. Pre-conception care of diabetes, congenital malformations, and spontaneous abortions. *Diabetes care.* 1996;19(5):514-41.
[26] Suhonen L, Hiilesmaa V, Teramo K. Glycaemic control during early pregnancy and fetal malformations in women with type I diabetes mellitus. *Diabetologia*. 2000;43(1):79-82.
[27] McMillan M, Porritt K, Kralik D, Costi L, Marshall H. Influenza vaccination during pregnancy: a systematic review of fetal death, spontaneous abortion, and congenital malformation safety outcomes. *Vaccine.* 2015;33(18):2108-17.
[28] Schellinger MM, Abernathy MP, Amerman B, May C, Foxlow LA, Carter AL, et al. Improved outcomes for hispanic women with gestational diabetes using the Centering Pregnancy© Group Prenatal Care Model. *Maternal and child health journal.* 2017;21(2):297-305.
[29] Casey BM, Duryea EL, Abbassi-Ghanavati M, Tudela CM, Shivvers SA, McIntire DD, et al. Glyburide in women with mild gestational diabetes: a randomized controlled trial. *Obstetrics & Gynecology.* 2015;126(2):303-9.
[30] Crowther CA, Hiller JE, Moss JR, McPhee AJ, Jeffries WS, Robinson JS. Effect of treatment of gestational diabetes mellitus on pregnancy outcomes. *New England Journal of Medicine*. 2005;352(24):2477-86.
[31] Sadeghi A, Hami J, Razavi S, Esfandiary E, Hejazi Z. The effect of diabetes mellitus on apoptosis in hippocampus: cellular and molecular aspects. *International journal of preventive medicine.* 2016;7.
[32] Diabetes IAo, Panel PSGC. International association of diabetes and pregnancy study groups recommendations on the diagnosis and classification of hyperglycemia in pregnancy. *Diabetes care.* 2010;33(3):676-82.
[33] Gabbe SG, Graves CR. Management of diabetes mellitus complicating pregnancy. *Obstetrics & Gynecology.* 2003;102(4):857-68.
[34] Bernasko J. Contemporary management of type 1 diabetes mellitus in pregnancy. *Obstetrical & gynecological survey.* 2004;59(8):628-36.
[35] Schwartz R, Teramo KA, editors. Effects of diabetic pregnancy on the fetus and newborn. *Seminars in perinatology;* 2000: Elsevier.

[36] Loffredo CA, Wilson PD, Ferencz C. Maternal diabetes: an independent risk factor for major cardiovascular malformations with increased mortality of affected infants. *Teratology.* 2001;64(2): 98-106.

[37] Meur S, Mann NP. Infant outcomes following diabetic pregnancies. *Paediatrics and Child Health.* 2007;17(6):217-22.

[38] Sells CJ, Robinson NM, Brown Z, Knopp RH. Long-term developmental follow-up of infants of diabetic mothers. *The Journal of pediatrics.* 1994;125(1):S9-S17.

[39] Loeken MR, editor Current perspectives on the causes of neural tube defects resulting from diabetic pregnancy. *American Journal of Medical Genetics Part C: Seminars in Medical Genetics;* 2005: Wiley Online Library.

[40] Dimitriu A, Russu G, Stamatin M, Jităreanu C, Streangă V. Clinical and developmental aspects of cardiac involvement in infant of diabetic mother. *Revista medico-chirurgicala a Societatii de Medici si Naturalisti din Iasi.* 2004;108(3):566-9.

[41] Manderson J, Mullan B, Patterson C, Hadden D, Traub A, McCance D. Cardiovascular and metabolic abnormalities in the offspring of diabetic pregnancy. *Diabetologia.* 2002;45(7):991-6.

[42] Hilvers PS, Rhodes LA, Gustafson RA, Castillo W. Tricuspid atresia and Tetralogy of fallot in an infant of a diabetic mother. *Pediatric cardiology.* 2009;30(3):382-4.

[43] Eriksson U, Dahlström E, Hellerström C. Diabetes in pregnancy: skeletal malformations in the offspring of diabetic rats after intermittent withdrawal of insulin in early gestation. *Diabetes.* 1983;32(12):1141-5.

[44] Passarge E, Lenz W. Syndrome of caudal regression in infants of diabetic mothers: observations of further cases. *Pediatrics.* 1966;37(4):672-5.

[45] Arizmendi J, Carmona Pertuz V, Colmenares A, Gómez Hoyos D, Palomo T. Gestational diabetes and neonatal complications. *Revista Med.* 2012;20(2):50-60.

[46] Viberti G, Bilous R, Mackintosh D, Bending J, Keen H. Long term correction of hyperglycaemia and progression of renal failure in

insulin dependent diabetes. *Br Med J (Clin Res Ed).* 1983;286 (6365):598-602.

[47] Soler N, Walsh C, Malins J. Congenital malformations in infants of diabetic mothers. *QJM: An International Journal of Medicine.* 1976;45(2):303-13.

[48] Sheffield JS, Butler-Koster EL, Casey BM, McIntire DD, Leveno KJ. Maternal diabetes mellitus and infant malformations. *Obstetrics & Gynecology.* 2002;100(5):925-30.

[49] Langer O, Conway DL. Level of glycemia and perinatal outcome in pregestational diabetes. *Journal of Maternal-Fetal Medicine.* 2000;9 (1):35-41.

[50] Hod M, Merlob P, Friedman S, Litwin A, Mor N, Rusecki Y, et al. Prevalence of minor congenital anomalies in newborns of diabetic mothers. *European Journal of Obstetrics and Gynecology and Reproductive Biology.* 1992;44(2):111-6.

[51] Evers IM, de Valk HW, Visser GH. Risk of complications of pregnancy in women with type 1 diabetes: nationwide prospective study in the Netherlands. *BMJ.* 2004;328(7445):915.

[52] Hami J, Karimi R, Haghir H, Gholamin M, Sadr-Nabavi A. Diabetes in pregnancy adversely affects the expression of glycogen synthase kinase-3β in the hippocampus of rat neonates. *Journal of Molecular Neuroscience.* 2015;57(2):273-81.

[53] Dall TM, Yang W, Halder P, Pang B, Massoudi M, Wintfeld N, et al. The economic burden of elevated blood glucose levels in 2012: diagnosed and undiagnosed diabetes, gestational diabetes mellitus, and prediabetes. *Diabetes care.* 2014;37(12):3172-9.

[54] Langer O, Levy J, Brustman L, Anyaegbunam A, Merkatz R, Divon M. Glycemic control in gestational diabetes mellitus-how tight is tight enough: small for gestational age versus large for gestational age? *American journal of obstetrics and gynecology.* 1989;161(3):646-53.

[55] Hami J, Shojae F, Vafaee-Nezhad S, Lotfi N, Kheradmand H, Haghir H. Some of the experimental and clinical aspects of the effects of the maternal diabetes on developing hippocampus. *World journal of diabetes.* 2015;6(3):412.

[56] Ornoy A. Neurobehavioral risks of SSRIs in pregnancy: Comparing human and animal data. *Reproductive Toxicology*. 2017;72:191-200.

[57] Kullmann S, Heni M, Hallschmid M, Fritsche A, Preissl H, Häring HU. Brain insulin resistance at the crossroads of metabolic and cognitive disorders in humans. *Physiological reviews*. 2016;96(4): 1169-209.

[58] Money K, Barke T, Serezani A, Gannon M, Garbett K, Aronoff D, et al. Gestational diabetes exacerbates maternal immune activation effects in the developing brain. *Molecular psychiatry*. 2017.

[59] Chandna A, Kuhlmann N, Bryce C, Greba Q, Campanucci V, Howland J. Chronic maternal hyperglycemia induced during mid-pregnancy in rats increases RAGE expression, augments hippocampal excitability, and alters behavior of the offspring. *Neuroscience*. 2015;303:241-60.

[60] Szkudelski T. The mechanism of alloxan and streptozotocin action in B cells of the rat pancreas. *Physiological research*. 2001;50(6): 537-46.

[61] Kinney B, Rabe M, Jensen R, Steger R. Maternal hyperglycemia leads to gender-dependent deficits in learning and memory in offspring. *Experimental Biology and Medicine*. 2003;228(2):152-9.

[62] Plagemann A, Harder T, Lindner R, Melchior K, Rake A, Rittel F, et al. Alterations of hypothalamic catecholamines in the newborn offspring of gestational diabetic mother rats. *Developmental Brain Research*. 1998;109(2):201-9.

[63] Copp AJ, Brook FA, Estibeiro JP, Shum AS, Cockroft DL. The embryonic development of mammalian neural tube defects. *Progress in neurobiology*. 1990;35(5):363-403.

[64] Greene ND, Copp AJ. Development of the vertebrate central nervous system: formation of the neural tube. *Prenatal diagnosis*. 2009;29(4):303-11.

[65] Karfunkel P. The mechanisms of neural tube formation. *International review of cytology*. 38: Elsevier; 1974. p. 245-71.

[66] Parchem RJ, Moore N, Fish JL, Parchem JG, Braga TT, Shenoy A, et al. miR-302 is required for timing of neural differentiation, neural tube closure, and embryonic viability. *Cell reports*. 2015;12(5):760-73.

[67] Dessaud E, McMahon AP, Briscoe J. Pattern formation in the vertebrate neural tube: a sonic hedgehog morphogen-regulated transcriptional network. *Development.* 2008;135(15):2489-503.

[68] Moore LL, Singer MR, Bradlee ML, Rothman KJ, Milunsky A. A prospective study of the risk of congenital defects associated with maternal obesity and diabetes mellitus. *Epidemiology.* 2000;11 (6):689-94.

[69] Salbaum JM, Kappen C. Neural tube defect genes and maternal diabetes during pregnancy. *Birth Defects Research Part A: Clinical and Molecular Teratology.* 2010;88(8):601-11.

[70] Dell'Edera D, Sarlo F, Allegretti A, Epifania A, Simone F, Lupo M, et al. Prevention of neural tube defects and maternal gestational diabetes through the inositol supplementation: preliminary results. *European review for medical and pharmacological sciences.* 2017;21:3305-11.

[71] Phelan SA, Ito M, Loeken MR. Neural tube defects in embryos of diabetic mice: role of the Pax-3 gene and apoptosis. *Diabetes.* 1997;46(7):1189-97.

[72] Meier P, Finch A, Evan G. Apoptosis in development. *Nature.* 2000;407(6805):796.

[73] Yu J, Mu J, Guo Q, Yang L, Zhang J, Liu Z, et al. Transcriptomic profile analysis of mouse neural tube development by RNA-Seq. *IUBMB lif*e. 2017;69(9):706-19.

[74] Sadler TW. *Langman's medical embryology:* Lippincott Williams & Wilkins; 2011.

[75] Wang L, Chang S, Wang Z, Wang S, Huo J, Ding G, et al. Altered GNAS imprinting due to folic acid deficiency contributes to poor embryo development and may lead to neural tube defects. *Oncotarget.* 2017;8(67):110797.

[76] Copp AJ, Greene ND. Genetics and development of neural tube defects. *The Journal of pathology.* 2010;220(2):217-30.

[77] Avagliano L, Tosi D, Scagliotti V, Gualtieri A, Gaston-Massuet C, Pistocchi A, et al. Cell death and cell proliferation in human spina bifida. *Birth Defects Research Part A: Clinical and Molecular Teratology.* 2016;106(2):104-13.

[78] Hami J, Sadr-Nabavi A, Sankian M, Balali-Mood M, Haghir H. The effects of maternal diabetes on expression of insulin-like growth factor-1 and insulin receptors in male developing rat hippocampus. *Brain Structure and Function.* 2013;218(1):73-84.

[79] Association AD. 12. Management of diabetes in pregnancy. *Diabetes care.* 2016;39(Supplement 1):S94-S8.

[80] Berry DC, Boggess K, Johnson QB. Management of pregnant women with type 2 diabetes mellitus and the consequences of fetal programming in their offspring. *Current diabetes reports.* 2016;16(5):36.

[81] Chen G, Sun W, Liang Y, Chen T, Guo W, Tian W. Maternal diabetes modulates offspring cell proliferation and apoptosis during odontogenesis via the TLR4/NF-κB signalling pathway. *Cell proliferation.* 2017;50(3).

[82] Lotfi N, Hami J, Hosseini M, Haghir D, Haghir H. Diabetes during pregnancy enhanced neuronal death in the hippocampus of rat offspring. *International Journal of Developmental Neuroscience.* 2016;51:28-35.

[83] Haghir H, Hami J, Lotfi N, Peyvandi M, Ghasemi S, Hosseini M. Expression of apoptosis-regulatory genes in the hippocampus of rat neonates born to mothers with diabetes. *Metabolic brain disease.* 2017;32(2):617-28.

[84] Ornoy A, Reece EA, Pavlinkova G, Kappen C, Miller RK. Effect of maternal diabetes on the embryo, fetus, and children: congenital anomalies, genetic and epigenetic changes and developmental outcomes. *Birth Defects Research Part C: Embryo Today: Reviews.* 2015;105(1):53-72.

[85] Zhao Z, Cao L, Reece EA. Formation of neurodegenerative aggresome and death-inducing signaling complex in maternal diabetes-induced neural tube defects. *Proceedings of the National Academy of Sciences.* 2017;114(17):4489-94.

[86] Gabbay-Benziv R, Reece EA, Wang F, Yang P. Birth defects in pregestational diabetes: Defect range, glycemic threshold and pathogenesis. *World journal of diabetes.* 2015;6(3):481.

[87] Zhong J, Xu C, Gabbay-Benziv R, Lin X, Yang P. Superoxide dismutase 2 overexpression alleviates maternal diabetes-induced neural tube defects, restores mitochondrial function and suppresses cellular stress in diabetic embryopathy. *Free Radical Biology and Medicine.* 2016;96:234-44.

[88] Ornoy A. Growth and neurodevelopmental outcome of children born to mothers with pregestational and gestational diabetes. *Pediatric endocrinology reviews: PER.* 2005;3(2):104-13.

[89] Ornoy A, Ratzon N, Greenbaum C, Peretz E, Soriano D, Dulitzky M. Neurobehaviour of school age children born to diabetic mothers. *Archives of Disease in Childhood-Fetal and Neonatal Edition.* 1998;79(2):F94-F9.

[90] Ornoy A, Wolf A, Ratzon N, Greenbaum C, Dulitzky M. Neurodevelopmental outcome at early school age of children born to mothers with gestational diabetes. *Archives of Disease in Childhood-Fetal and Neonatal Edition.* 1999;81(1):F10-F4.

[91] Fraser A, Almqvist C, Larsson H, Långström N, Lawlor DA. Maternal diabetes in pregnancy and offspring cognitive ability: sibling study with 723,775 men from 579,857 families. *Diabetologia.* 2014;57 (1):102-9.

[92] Ornoy A, Ratzon N, Greenbaum C, Wolf A, Dulitzky M. School-age children born to diabetic mothers and to mothers with gestational diabetes exhibit a high rate of inattention and fine and gross motor impairment. *Journal of Pediatric Endocrinology and Metabolism.* 2001;14(Supplement):681-90.

[93] Babiker O. Long-term effects of maternal diabetes on their offspring development and behaviours. *Sudanese J Ped.* 2007;8:133-46.

[94] Rizzo T, Metzger BE, Burns WJ, Burns K. Correlations between antepartum maternal metabolism and intelligence of offspring. *New England Journal of Medicine.* 1991;325(13):911-6.

[95] Haghir H, Nomani H, Sankian M, Kheradmand H, Hami J. Sexual dimorphism in expression of insulin and insulin-like growth factor-I receptors in developing rat cerebellum. *Cellular and molecular neurobiology.* 2013;33(3):369-77.

[96] Hami J, Sadr-Nabavi A, Sankian M, Haghir H. Sex differences and left–right asymmetries in expression of insulin and insulin-like growth factor-1 receptors in developing rat hippocampus. *Brain Structure and Function.* 2012;217(2):293-302.

[97] Golalipour M, Kafshgiri SK, Ghafari S. Gestational diabetes induced neuronal loss in CA1 and CA3 subfields of rat hippocampus in early postnatal life. *Folia morphologica.* 2012;71(2):71-7.

[98] Kafshgiri SK, Ghafari S, Golalipour MJ. Gestational diabetes induces neuronal loss in dentate gyrus in rat offspring. *Journal of Neurological Sciences.* 2014;31(2):316-24.

[99] Tehranipour M, Khakzad M. Effect of maternal diabetes on hippocampus neuronal density in neonatal rats. *J Biol Sci.* 2008;6:1027-32.

[100] Fu J, Tay S, Ling E, Dheen S. High glucose alters the expression of genes involved in proliferation and cell-fate specification of embryonic neural stem cells. *Diabetologia.* 2006;49(5):1027-38.

[101] Gao Q, Gao YM. Hyperglycemic condition disturbs the proliferation and cell death of neural progenitors in mouse embryonic spinal cord. *International Journal of Developmental Neuroscience.* 2007;25(6): 349-57.

[102] Hami J, Vafaei-Nezhad S, Haghir D, Haghir H. Insulin-like growth factor-1 receptor is differentially distributed in developing cerebellar cortex of rats born to diabetic mothers. *Journal of Molecular Neuroscience.* 2016;58(2):221-32.

[103] Hami J, Kheradmand H, Haghir H. Gender differences and lateralization in the distribution pattern of insulin-like growth factor-1 receptor in developing rat hippocampus: an immunohistochemical study. *Cellular and molecular neurobiology.* 2014;34(2):215-26.

[104] Hsieh J, Aimone JB, Kaspar BK, Kuwabara T, Nakashima K, Gage FH. IGF-I instructs multipotent adult neural progenitor cells to become oligodendrocytes. *The Journal of cell biology.* 2004;164(1):111-22.

[105] Haghir H, Sankian M, Kheradmand H, Hami J. The effects of induced type-I diabetes on developmental regulation of insulin & insulin like

growth factor-1 (IGF-1) receptors in the cerebellum of rat neonates. *Metabolic brain disease.* 2013;28(3):397-410.

[106] Hernández-Fonseca JP, Rincón J, Pedreañez A, Viera N, Arcaya JL, Carrizo E, et al. Structural and ultrastructural analysis of cerebral cortex, cerebellum, and hypothalamus from diabetic rats. *Experimental Diabetes Research.* 2009;2009.

[107] Hami J, Vafaei-nezhad S, Ghaemi K, Sadeghi A, Ivar G, Shojae F, et al. Stereological study of the effects of maternal diabetes on cerebellar cortex development in rat. *Metabolic brain disease.* 2016;31(3):643-52.

[108] Khaksar Z, Jelodar G, Hematian H. Cerebrum malformation in offspring of diabetic mothers. *Comparative Clinical Pathology.* 2012;21 (5):699-703.

[109] Khaksar Z, Jelodar G, Hematian H. *Morphometric study of cerebrum in fetuses of diabetic mothers.* 2011.

[110] Vuong B, Odero G, Rozbacher S, Stevenson M, Kereliuk SM, Pereira TJ, et al. Exposure to gestational diabetes mellitus induces neuroinflammation, derangement of hippocampal neurons, and cognitive changes in rat offspring. *Journal of neuroinflammation.* 2017; 14(1):80.

[111] Hami J, Vafaei-Nezhad S, Ivar G, Sadeghi A, Ghaemi K, Mostafavizadeh M, et al. Altered expression and localization of synaptophysin in developing cerebellar cortex of neonatal rats due to maternal diabetes mellitus. *Metabolic brain disease.* 2016;31(6): 1369-80.

[112] Hami J, Vafaei-Nezhad S, Sadeghi A, Ghaemi K, Taheri MMH, Fereidouni M, et al. Synaptogenesis in the cerebellum of offspring born to diabetic mothers. *Journal of pediatric neurosciences.* 2017;12(3):215.

[113] Brooks V. Comment: On functions of the" cerebellar circuit" in movement control. *Canadian journal of physiology and pharmacology.* 1981;59(7):776-8.

[114] Eccles JC. Physiology of motor control in man. *Stereotactic and Functional Neurosurgery.* 1981;44(1-3):5-15.

[115] Beaton A, Mariën P. *Language, cognition and the cerebellum: grappling with an enigma. cortex.* 2010;46(7):811-20.

[116] Bugalho P, Correa B, Viana-Baptista M. Role of the cerebellum in cognitive and behavioural control: scientific basis and investigation models. *Acta medica portuguesa.* 2006;19(3):257-67.

[117] Diamond A. Close interrelation of motor development and cognitive development and of the cerebellum and prefrontal cortex. *Child development.* 2000;71(1):44-56.

[118] Dolan R. A cognitive affective role for the cerebellum. *Brain: a journal of neurology.* 1998;121(4):545-6.

[119] Hayter A, Langdon D, Ramnani N. Cerebellar contributions to working memory. *Neuroimage.* 2007;36(3):943-54.

[120] Schmahmann JD, Sherman JC. The cerebellar cognitive affective syndrome. *Brain: a journal of neurology.* 1998;121(4):561-79.

[121] Schutter DJ, van Honk J. An electrophysiological link between the cerebellum, cognition and emotion: frontal theta EEG activity to single-pulse cerebellar TMS. *Neuroimage.* 2006;33(4):1227-31.

[122] Turner BM, Paradiso S, Marvel CL, Pierson R, Ponto LLB, Hichwa RD, et al. The cerebellum and emotional experience. *Neuropsychologia.* 2007;45(6):1331-41.

[123] Marvel CL, Desmond JE. Functional topography of the cerebellum in verbal working memory. *Neuropsychology review.* 2010;20(3):271-9.

[124] Desmond JE, Fiez JA. Neuroimaging studies of the cerebellum: language, learning and memory. *Trends in cognitive sciences.* 1998;2(9):355-62.

[125] Altman J. Postnatal development of the cerebellar cortex in the rat. I. The external germinal layer and the transitional molecular layer. *Journal of Comparative Neurology.* 1972;145(3):353-97.

[126] Altman J, Bayer SA. *Development of the cerebellar system: in relation to its evolution, structure, and functions*: CRC; 1997.

[127] Altman J, Winfree AT. Postnatal development of the cerebellar cortex in the rat: V. Spatial organization of Purkinje cell perikarya. *Journal of Comparative Neurology.* 1977;171(1):1-16.

[128] Butts T, Green MJ, Wingate RJ. Development of the cerebellum: simple steps to make a 'little brain'. *Development.* 2014;141(21): 4031-41.

[129] de Zeeuw CI, Strata P, Voogd J. *The cerebellum: from structure to control:* Elsevier Science; 1997.

[130] Hans J, Lammens M. Development of the human cerebellum and its disorders. *Clinics in perinatology.* 2009;36(3):513-30.

[131] Hans J, Lammens M, Wesseling P, Hori A. Development and developmental disorders of the human cerebellum. *Clinical neuroembryology:* Springer; 2014. p. 371-420.

[132] Thach WT, Goodkin H, Keating J. The cerebellum and the adaptive coordination of movement. *Annual review of neuroscience.* 1992;15(1):403-42.

[133] Petzoldt AG, Sigrist SJ. Synaptogenesis. *Current Biology.* 2014;24 (22):R1076-R80.

[134] Yamaguchi Y. Glycobiology of the synapse: the role of glycans in the formation, maturation, and modulation of synapses. *Biochimica et Biophysica Acta (BBA)-General Subjects.* 2002;1573(3):369-76.

[135] Sanes J. The formation and regeneration of synapses. *The principles of neuroscience.* 2000:1087-114.

[136] Poon VYN, Choi S, Park M. Growth factors in synaptic function. *Frontiers in synaptic neuroscience.* 2013;5:6.

[137] Garner CC, Shen K. Structure and function of vertebrate and invertebrate active zones. *Structural and Functional Organization of the Synapse:* Springer; 2008. p. 63-89.

[138] Schoch S, Gundelfinger ED. Molecular organization of the presynaptic active zone. *Cell and tissue research.* 2006;326(2):379-91.

[139] Montgomery J, Zamorano P, Garner C. MAGUKs in synapse assembly and function: an emerging view. *Cellular and Molecular Life Sciences CMLS.* 2004;61(7-8):911-29.

[140] Vafaei-Nezhad S, Hami J, Sadeghi A, Ghaemi K, Hosseini M, Abedini M, et al. The impacts of diabetes in pregnancy on hippocampal synaptogenesis in rat neonates. *Neuroscience.* 2016;318:122-33.

[141] Waites CL, Craig AM, Garner CC. Mechanisms of vertebrate synaptogenesis. *Annu Rev Neurosci.* 2005;28:251-74.

[142] Garner CC, Zhai RG, Gundelfinger ED, Ziv NE. Molecular mechanisms of CNS synaptogenesis. *Trends in neurosciences.* 2002;25(5):243-50.

[143] Schikorski T, Stevens CF. Morphological correlates of functionally defined synaptic vesicle populations. *Nature neuroscience.* 2001;4 (4):391.

[144] Bennett MK, Calakos N, Scheller RH. Syntaxin: a synaptic protein implicated in docking of synaptic vesicles at presynaptic active zones. *Science.* 1992;257(5067):255-9.

[145] Luján R, Roberts JDB, Shigemoto R, Ohishi H, Somogyi P. Differential plasma membrane distribution of metabotropic glutamate receptors mGluR1α, mGluR2 and mGluR5, relative to neurotransmitter release sites. *Journal of chemical neuroanatomy.* 1997;13(4):219-41.

[146] Galarreta M, Hestrin S. Electrical and chemical synapses among parvalbumin fast-spiking GABAergic interneurons in adult mouse neocortex. *Proceedings of the National Academy of Sciences.* 2002;99(19):12438-43.

[147] Pereda AE. Electrical synapses and their functional interactions with chemical synapses. *Nature Reviews Neuroscience.* 2014;15(4):250.

[148] DeFelipe J, Fariñas I. The pyramidal neuron of the cerebral cortex: morphological and chemical characteristics of the synaptic inputs. *Progress in neurobiology.* 1992;39(6):563-607.

[149] Davis EK. *Regulation of hippocampal synapse formation and specificity*: UC San Diego; 2008.

[150] Sudhof TC. The synaptic vesicle cycle. *Annual review of neuroscience.* 2004;27:509.

[151] Südhof TC. The synaptic vesicle cycle: a cascade of protein–protein interactions. *Nature.* 1995;375(6533):645.

[152] Schweizer FE, Ryan TA. The synaptic vesicle: cycle of exocytosis and endocytosis. *Current opinion in neurobiology.* 2006;16(3):298-304.

[153] Zhai RG, Vardinon-Friedman H, Cases-Langhoff C, Becker B, Gundelfinger ED, Ziv NE, et al. Assembling the presynaptic active

zone: a characterization of an active zone precursor vesicle. *Neuron.* 2001;29(1):131-43.

[154] Han Y, Kaeser PS, Südhof TC, Schneggenburger R. RIM determines Ca2+ channel density and vesicle docking at the presynaptic active zone. *Neuron.* 2011;69(2):304-16.

[155] Chen G, Wu X, Tuncdemir S. Cell adhesion and synaptogenesis. *Sheng li xue bao:[Acta physiologica Sinica].* 2007;59(6):697-706.

[156] Zenisek D, Steyer J, Almers W. Transport, capture and exocytosis of single synaptic vesicles at active zones. *Nature.* 2000;406(6798):849.

[157] Zhu P, Thureson-Klein Å, Klein R. Exocytosis from large dense cored vesicles outside the active synaptic zones of terminals within the trigeminal subnucleus caudalis: a possible mechanism for neuropeptide release. *Neuroscience.* 1986;19(1):43-54.

[158] Michel K, Müller JA, Oprişoreanu AM, Schoch S. The presynaptic active zone: A dynamic scaffold that regulates synaptic efficacy. *Experimental cell research.* 2015;335(2):157-64.

[159] Davletov B, Montecucco C. Lipid function at synapses. *Current opinion in neurobiology.* 2010;20(5):543-9.

[160] Gincel D, Shoshan-Barmatz V. The synaptic vesicle protein synaptophysin: purification and characterization of its channel activity. *Biophysical journal.* 2002;83(6):3223-9.

[161] Dityatev A, *El-Husseini A. Molecular mechanisms of synaptogenesis:* Springer Science & Business Media; 2006.

[162] Klingauf J, Kavalali ET, Tsien RW. Kinetics and regulation of fast endocytosis at hippocampal synapses. *Nature.* 1998;394(6693):581.

[163] Huang LC, Thorne PR, Housley GD, Montgomery JM. Spatiotemporal definition of neurite outgrowth, refinement and retraction in the developing mouse cochlea. *Development.* 2007;134(16):2925-33.

[164] Sze CI, Troncoso JC, Kawas C, Mouton P, Price DL, Martin LJ. Loss of the presynaptic vesicle protein synaptophysin in hippocampus correlates with cognitive decline in Alzheimer disease. *Journal of Neuropathology & Experimental Neurology.* 1997;56(8):933-44.

[165] Terry RD, Masliah E, Salmon DP, Butters N, DeTeresa R, Hill R, et al. Physical basis of cognitive alterations in Alzheimer's disease:

synapse loss is the major correlate of cognitive impairment. *Annals of neurology*. 1991;30(4):572-80.

[166] Smith TD, Adams MM, Gallagher M, Morrison JH, Rapp PR. Circuit-specific alterations in hippocampal synaptophysin immunoreactivity predict spatial learning impairment in aged rats. *Journal of Neuroscience*. 2000;20(17):6587-93.

[167] Kvartsberg H, Duits FH, Ingelsson M, Andreasen N, Öhrfelt A, Andersson K, et al. Cerebrospinal fluid levels of the synaptic protein neurogranin correlates with cognitive decline in prodromal Alzheimer's disease. *Alzheimer's & dementia: the journal of the Alzheimer's Association*. 2015;11(10):1180-90.

[168] Lin MZ, Schnitzer MJ. Genetically encoded indicators of neuronal activity. *Nature neuroscience*. 2016;19(9):1142.

[169] Pulido C, Trigo FF, Llano I, Marty A. Vesicular release statistics and unitary postsynaptic current at single GABAergic synapses. *Neuron*. 2015;85(1):159-72.

[170] Wiedenmann B, Franke WW, Kuhn C, Moll R, Gould VE. Synaptophysin: a marker protein for neuroendocrine cells and neoplasms. *Proceedings of the National Academy of Sciences*. 1986;83(10):3500-4.

[171] Arthur CP, Stowell MH. Structure of synaptophysin: a hexameric MARVEL-domain channel protein. *Structure*. 2007;15(6):707-14.

[172] Jahn R, Schiebler W, Ouimet C, Greengard P. A 38,000-dalton membrane protein (p38) present in synaptic vesicles. *Proceedings of the National Academy of Sciences*. 1985;82(12):4137-41.

[173] Johnston P, Südhof T. The multisubunit structure of synaptophysin. Relationship between disulfide bonding and homo-oligomerization. *Journal of Biological Chemistry*. 1990;265(15):8869-73.

[174] Gordon SL, Harper CB, Smillie KJ, Cousin MA. A fine balance of synaptophysin levels underlies efficient retrieval of synaptobrevin II to synaptic vesicles. *PloS one*. 2016;11(2):e0149457.

[175] Valtorta F, Pennuto M, Bonanomi D, Benfenati F. Synaptophysin: leading actor or walk-on role in synaptic vesicle exocytosis? *Bioessays*. 2004;26(4):445-53.

[176] Kwon SE, Chapman ER. Synaptophysin regulates the kinetics of synaptic vesicle endocytosis in central neurons. *Neuron.* 2011; 70(5):847-54.

[177] Zhang B, Koh YH, Beckstead RB, Budnik V, Ganetzky B, Bellen HJ. Synaptic vesicle size and number are regulated by a clathrin adaptor protein required for endocytosis. *Neuron.* 1998;21(6):1465-75.

[178] Edelmann L, Hanson P, Chapman E, Jahn R. Synaptobrevin binding to synaptophysin: a potential mechanism for controlling the exocytotic fusion machine. *The EMBO journal.* 1995;14(2):224-31.

[179] Eshkind LG, Leube RE. Mice lacking synaptophysin reproduce and form typical synaptic vesicles. *Cell and tissue research.* 1995;282 (3):423-33.

[180] Pyeon HJ, Lee YI. Differential expression levels of synaptophysin through developmental stages in hippocampal region of mouse brain. *Anatomy & cell biology.* 2012;45(2):97-102.

[181] Alladi P, Wadhwa S, Singh N. Effect of prenatal auditory enrichment on developmental expression of synaptophysin and syntaxin 1 in chick brainstem auditory nuclei. *Neuroscience.* 2002;114(3):577-90.

[182] Janz R, Südhof TC, Hammer RE, Unni V, Siegelbaum SA, Bolshakov VY. Essential roles in synaptic plasticity for synaptogyrin I and synaptophysin I. *Neuron.* 1999;24(3):687-700.

[183] Ozcelik T, Lafreniere R, Archer 3rd B, Johnston P, Willard H, Francke U, et al. Synaptophysin: structure of the human gene and assignment to the X chromosome in man and mouse. *American journal of human genetics.* 1990;47(3):551.

[184] McMahon HT, Bolshakov VY, Janz R, Hammer RE, Siegelbaum SA, Südhof TC. Synaptophysin, a major synaptic vesicle protein, is not essential for neurotransmitter release. *Proceedings of the National Academy of Sciences.* 1996;93(10):4760-4.

[185] Li L, Tasic B, Micheva KD, Ivanov VM, Spletter ML, Smith SJ, et al. Visualizing the distribution of synapses from individual neurons in the mouse brain. *PloS one.* 2010;5(7):e11503.

[186] Elibol-Can B, Kilic E, Yuruker S, Jakubowska-Dogru E. Investigation into the effects of prenatal alcohol exposure on postnatal spine development and expression of synaptophysin and PSD95 in rat

hippocampus. *International Journal of Developmental Neuroscience.* 2014;33:106-14.

[187] Heinonen O, Soininen H, Sorvari H, Kosunen O, Palja L, Koivisto E, et al. Loss of synaptophysin-like immunoreactivity in the hippocampal formation is an early phenomenon in Alzheimer's disease. *Neuroscience.* 1995;64(2):375-84.

[188] Joca SR, Guimarães FS, Del-Bel E. Inhibition of nitric oxide synthase increases synaptophysin mRNA expression in the hippocampal formation of rats. *Neuroscience letters.* 2007;421(1):72-6.

[189] Masliah E, Terry RD, DeTeresa RM, Hansen LA. Immunohistochemical quantification of the synapse-related protein synaptophysin in Alzheimer disease. *Neuroscience letters.* 1989;103(2):234-9.

[190] Zhan SS, Beyreuther K, Schmitt H. Quantitative Assessment of the Synaptophysin Immuno-Reactivity of the Cortical Neuropil in Various Neurodegenerative Disorderswith Dementia. *Dementia and Geriatric Cognitive Disorders.* 1993;4(2):66-74.

[191] Thome J, Pesold B, Baader M, Hu M, Gewirtz JC, Duman RS, et al. Stress differentially regulates synaptophysin and synaptotagmin expression in hippocampus. *Biological psychiatry.* 2001;50(10): 809-12.

[192] Robles MC, Campoy C, Fernandez LG, Lopez-Pedrosa JM, Rueda R, Martin MJ. Maternal diabetes and cognitive performance in the offspring: a systematic review and meta-analysis. *PLoS One.* 2015;10(11):e0142583.

[193] Li M, Fallin MD, Riley A, Landa R, Walker SO, Silverstein M, et al. The association of maternal obesity and diabetes with autism and other developmental disabilities. *Pediatrics.* 2016;137(2):e20152206.

[194] Van Lieshout RJ, Voruganti LP. Diabetes mellitus during pregnancy and increased risk of schizophrenia in offspring: a review of the evidence and putative mechanisms. *Journal of psychiatry & neuroscience: JPN.* 2008;33(5):395.

[195] Daraki V, Roumeliotaki T, Koutra K, Georgiou V, Kampouri M, Kyriklaki A, et al. Effect of parental obesity and gestational diabetes on child neuropsychological and behavioral development at 4 years of

age: the Rhea mother–child cohort, Crete, Greece. *European Child & Adolescent Psychiatry*. 2017;26(6):703-14.

[196] DeBoer T, Wewerka S, Bauer PJ, Georgieff MK, Nelson CA. Explicit memory performance in infants of diabetic mothers at 1 year of age. *Developmental Medicine & Child Neurology*. 2005;47(8):525-31.

[197] Xiang AH, Wang X, Martinez MP, Walthall JC, Curry ES, Page K, et al. Association of maternal diabetes with autism in offspring. *JAMA*. 2015;313(14):1425-34.

[198] Rizzo T, Freinkel N, Metzger BE, Hatcher R, Burns WJ, Barglow P. Correlations between antepartum maternal metabolism and newborn behavior. *American journal of obstetrics and gynecology*. 1990;163 (5):1458-64.

[199] Hami J, Hosseini M, Ivar G, Vafaei-Nezhad S, Keivan M. Cognitive Function in Offspring of Mothers with Gestational Diabetes–The Role of Insulin receptor. *MOJ Anat & Physiol*. 2016;2(7):00072.

[200] Towner D, Kjos SL, Leung B, Montoro MM, Xiang A, Mestman JH, et al. Congenital Malformations in Pregnancies Complicated by NIDDM: Increased risk from poor maternal metabolic control but not from exposure to sulfonylurea drugs. *Diabetes Care*. 1995;18(11): 1446-51.

[201] Group NDD. Classification and diagnosis of diabetes mellitus and other categories of glucose intolerance. *Diabetes*. 1979;28(12): 1039-57.

[202] Chen CH, Adam PA, Laskowski DE, McCann ML, Schwartz R. The plasma free fatty acid composition and blood glucose of normal and diabetic pregnant women and of their newborns. *Pediatrics*. 1965;36(6):843-55.

[203] De Vivo DC, Trifiletti RR, Jacobson RI, Ronen GM, Behmand RA, Harik SI. Defective glucose transport across the blood-brain barrier as a cause of persistent hypoglycorrhachia, seizures, and developmental delay. *New England Journal of Medicine*. 1991;325(10):703-9.

[204] Van Assche FA, Holemans K, Aerts L. Long-term consequences for offspring of diabetes during pregnancy. *British medical bulletin*. 2001;60(1):173-82.

[205] Aerts L, Holemans K, Van Assche FA. Maternal diabetes during pregnancy: consequences for the offspring. *Diabetes/Metabolism Research and Reviews.* 1990;6(3):147-67.

[206] Di Cianni G, Miccoli R, Volpe L, Lencioni C, Del Prato S. Intermediate metabolism in normal pregnancy and in gestational diabetes. *Diabetes/metabolism research and reviews.* 2003;19(4): 259-70.

[207] Philipps A, Porte P, Stabinsky S, Rosenkrantz T, Raye J. Effects of chronic fetal hyperglycemia upon oxygen consumption in the ovine uterus and conceptus. *The Journal of clinical investigation.* 1984;74(1):279-86.

[208] Anderson MS, Flowers-Ziegler J, Das UG, Hay Jr WW, Devaskar SU. Glucose transporter protein responses to selective hyperglycemia or hyperinsulinemia in fetal sheep. *American Journal of Physiology-Regulatory, Integrative and Comparative Physiology.* 2001;281 (5):R1545-R52.

[209] Scholtens DM, Bain JR, Reisetter AC, Muehlbauer MJ, Nodzenski M, Stevens RD, et al. Metabolic networks and metabolites underlie associations between maternal glucose during pregnancy and newborn size at birth. *Diabetes.* 2016:db151748.

[210] Eriksson UJ, Wentzel P. The status of diabetic embryopathy. *Upsala journal of medical sciences.* 2016;121(2):96-112.

[211] Moazzen H, Lu X, Liu M, Feng Q. Pregestational diabetes induces fetal coronary artery malformation via reactive oxygen species signaling. *Diabetes.* 2015;64(4):1431-43.

[212] Damasceno DC, Netto A, Iessi I, Gallego F, Corvino S, Dallaqua B, et al. Streptozotocin-induced diabetes models: pathophysiological mechanisms and fetal outcomes. *BioMed Research International.* 2014.

[213] Yang P, Reece EA, Wang F, Gabbay-Benziv R. Decoding the oxidative stress hypothesis in diabetic embryopathy through proapoptotic kinase signaling. *American Journal of Obstetrics & Gynecology.* 2015;212(5):569-79.

[214] Moreli JB, Santos JH, Lorenzon-Ojea AR, Corrêa-Silva S, Fortunato RS, Rocha CR, et al. Hyperglycemia differentially affects maternal

and fetal DNA integrity and DNA damage response. *International journal of biological sciences.* 2016;12(4):466.

[215] Casanueva E, Viteri FE. Iron and oxidative stress in pregnancy. *The Journal of nutrition.* 2003;133(5):1700S-8S.

[216] Swaminathan S, Fonseca VA, Alam MG, Shah SV. The role of iron in diabetes and its complications. *Diabetes care.* 2007;30(7):1926-33.

[217] Scholl TO. Iron status during pregnancy: setting the stage for mother and infant–. *The American journal of clinical nutrition.* 2005;81 (5):1218S-22S.

[218] Georgieff MK. Long-term brain and behavioral consequences of early iron deficiency. *Nutrition reviews.* 2011;69(s1).

[219] Armony-Sivan R, Eidelman AI, Lanir A, Sredni D, Yehuda S. Iron status and neurobehavioral development of premature infants. *Journal of perinatology.* 2004;24(12):757.

[220] Lozoff B, Jimenez E, Wolf AW. Long-term developmental outcome of infants with iron deficiency. *New England journal of medicine.* 1991;325(10):687-94.

[221] Rao R, Tkac I, Townsend EL, Gruetter R, Georgieff MK. Perinatal iron deficiency alters the neurochemical profile of the developing rat hippocampus. *The Journal of nutrition.* 2003;133(10):3215-21.

[222] Beard J. Iron Deficiency Alters Brain Development and Functioning, 2. *The Journal of nutrition.* 2003;133(5):1468S-72S.

[223] Lucas MJ, Leveno KJ, Williams ML, Raskin P, Whalley PJ. Early pregnancy glycosylated hemoglobin, severity of diabetes, and fetal malformations. *American Journal of Obstetrics & Gynecology.* 1989; 161(2):426-31.

[224] Silverman BL, Metzger BE, Cho NH, Loeb CA. Impaired glucose tolerance in adolescent offspring of diabetic mothers: relationship to fetal hyperinsulinism. *Diabetes care.* 1995;18(5):611-7.

[225] Longo LD. Maternal Complications of Pregnancy that Affect Fetal Development. *The Rise of Fetal and Neonatal Physiology:* Springer; 2018. p. 281-364.

[226] Coughlan M, Oliva K, Georgiou H, Permezel J, Rice G. Glucose-induced release of tumour necrosis factor-alpha from human placental

and adipose tissues in gestational diabetes mellitus. *Diabetic Medicine.* 2001;18(11):921-7.

[227] Sampson MJ, Gopaul N, Davies IR, Hughes DA, Carrier MJ. Plasma F2 isoprostanes: direct evidence of increased free radical damage during acute hyperglycemia in type 2 diabetes. *Diabetes care.* 2002;25(3):537-41.

[228] Eriksson UJ, Borg LH. Diabetes and embryonic malformations: role of substrate-induced free-oxygen radical production for dysmorphogenesis in cultured rat embryos. *Diabetes.* 1993;42(3): 411-9.

[229] Lee AT, Reis D, Eriksson UJ. Hyperglycemia-induced embryonic dysmorphogenesis correlates with genomic DNA mutation frequency in vitro and in vivo. *Diabetes.* 1999;48(2):371-6.

In: Development of the Cerebellum
Editor: Severina Fabbri
ISBN: 978-1-53614-317-1

Chapter 3

THE SPACES WHERE ADDICTION ACTS: FOCUS ON DRUG-INDUCED MOLECULAR AND CELLULAR CHANGES IN THE CEREBELLUM

Saeed Solouki[1,*] and Hossein Soltanloo[2]
[1]Department of Biomedical Engineering,
Human Motor Control and Computational Neuroscience Lab,
University of Tehran, Tehran, Iran
[2]Department of Artificial Intelligence,
Association for Computing Machinery Community,
University of Tehran, Tehran, Iran

ABSTRACT

Acute and chronic opioid consumption causes significant impairments in motor functioning, suggest an involvement of cerebellar circuits in fine tuning of movement patterns. Increasing evidence has involved the cerebellum in addictive behavior. We aimed on cellular and molecular

---

* Corresponding Author Email: saidsolooki@gmail.com, s.solouki@ut.ac.ir.

targets in the cerebellum where opioids can induce or alter mechanisms of neuroplasticity that may contribute to the development of an addictive behavioral pattern. Also, we investigated the consequences of repetitive drug administration on cerebellar synaptic efficiency. Insight into the neural mechanisms underlying these impairments has largely stemmed from clinical animal studies. The results of these studies agree to relevant participation of the cerebellum in the functional systems underlying drug-induced long-term memory and the perseverative behavioral phenotype. The molecular and neuronal actions of addictive drugs in the cerebellum involve long-term adaptive changes in receptors, neurotransmitters and intracellular signaling transduction pathways that may lead to the reorganization of cerebellar micro complexes or recreation of new domains of attraction. As a part of this functional reorganization, drug-induced cerebellar hyper-responsiveness appears to be central in reducing the influence of executive control of the prefrontal cortex on behavior and aiding the transition to an automatic mode of control. As a result, it can be expected that improved understanding of the neural mechanisms affected by drug addiction has the potential to advance the diagnoses, treatment or even prevention of behavioral disorders.

Keywords: cerebellar plasticity, drug addiction, ethanol, cocaine, morphine, endocannabinoids, amphetamine, sensitization, conditioning

1. INTRODUCTION

The negative impacts of excessive drug consumption often lead to long-term learning and memory impairments [1]. Over the past decade, a convergence of clinical and basic investigations of addictive substances has implicated the cerebellum in addiction. Human neuroimaging studies estimate that the extent of the malfunction caused by chronic application of addictive drugs goes beyond the sphere of motor control and involves non-motor functions related to cognitive skills [2]. The behavioral changes in such non-motor functions provide a suitable bed for evaluating the potential role of the cerebellum in addiction. In brief, the cerebellum receives extensive direct and indirect afferent input from prefrontal and association cortices in the cerebrum. Lesions to the posterior cerebellar hemispheres can lead to cerebellar cognitive affective syndrome, which features higher-level deficits beyond motor planning and execution [2, 3].

In this review, we outline exemplary animal and human findings that guide our current understanding of how chronic drug administration alters neural structure and function of the cerebellum. We mainly focus on reviewing evidence that involves the cerebellum in addictive behavior. First, we aimed on molecular and cellular targets in the cerebellum where addictive drugs can act and induce mechanisms of neuroplasticity that may contribute to the development of an addictive pattern of behavior. Then, we analyze behavioral consequences of repetitive drug administration that result from activity-dependent changes in the efficacy of cerebellar synapses. Finally, we describe common hypotheses that underlie drug-induced structural and functional changes in the cerebellum.

2. Gross Neuroanatomy of the Cerebellum

The human cerebellum contains the most number of neurons in the brain [4]. It consists of two hemispheres connected by a midline structure, the vermis. The cerebellar surface appears undulated in the rostrocaudal orientation, which results from the presence of transverse fissures. Some of these fissures extend to the lateral border of the cerebellum. The arrangement of fissures led to the recognition of three different lobes, which in turn are further subdivided into 10 lobules: The anterior lobe contains lobules I–V, the posterior lobe contains lobules VI–IX and the flocculonodular lobe contains lobule X (Figure 1a). Like the cerebral cortex, the cerebellum has an outer cortical layer made up of gray matter, and with an inner layer of white matter scaffolding [5]. The cerebellar peduncles form a thick trunk of white matter that connects the cerebellum to the brainstem. The cerebellar cortex has a highly foliated structure consisting of three distinct layers (molecular, Purkinje cell and granular layers) (Figure 1b). Purkinje cells are inhibitory neurons that project to the deep cerebellar neurons and regulate their efferent signal output to the brainstem and cerebral cortex. The cerebellum receives two major input from the inferior olive and the pontine nuclei, through the climbing fibers and mossy fiber pathways, respectively (Figure 1c).

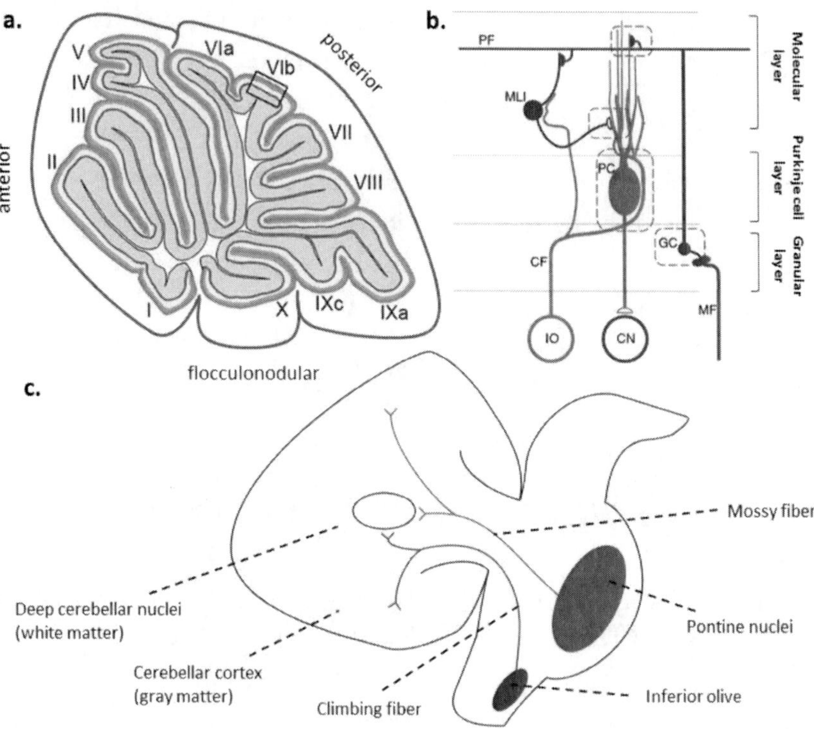

Figure 1. Cerebellar anatomy. (a) Schematic representation of the cerebellar lobules (b) Cortical layers in the cerebellum (c) Sagittal view highlighting the major afferent pathways into the cerebellum. Mossy fibers project to granule cells in the cerebellar cortex, and send collaterals to the deep cerebellar nuclei. Climbing fibers extend to Purkinje cells, and also have collateral projections to deep cerebellar nuclei. The axons of the deep cerebellar nuclei form the primary output channels away from the cerebellum and to the brainstem and cerebral cortex.

The functional unit of the cerebellar cortex is named microzones, that refers a corticonuclear arrangement. Microzones themselves form part of a larger entity called multizonal microcomplex. Each microcomplex is involved in a functional network to different parts of the cerebral cortex and spinal cord [5, 6], the thalamus [5], the septo-hippocampal complex and the amygdala [6]. All these anatomical pathways locate the cerebellum within the functional systems where addictive drugs can act and produce their behavioral effects. In following sections, we describe the synaptic organization in the cerebellum and how molecular targets in the cerebellar synapses are affected by addictive drugs.

3. Different Forms of Synaptic Plasticity in the Cerebellum

Neurons in the cerebellar cortex and neurons in cerebellar and vestibular nuclei show various forms of synaptic and intrinsic plasticity [7], and neurons in both regions are innervated by axons from the mossy fibre and climbing fibre system. This raises the possibility that the various forms of plasticity induced in the cerebellar cortex and nuclei are not independent but are finely regulated in a coordinated manner [7, 8], and that some of the memories that are formed in the cerebellar cortex are also ultimately consolidated and stored in the cerebellar and vestibular nuclei [9]. The cerebellar cortex has two main afferent pathways (Figure 2). Mossy fiber afferents are derived from various brainstem nuclei. A single mossy fibre can divide across different folia into multiple branches, each of which provides multiple rosettes; a single mossy fibre rosette provides excitatory input to tens of granule cells within a glomerulus (Figure 2). The granular cells, in turn, project to the molecular layer and excite the Purkinje cells. Within the glomerulus, the dendrites of granular cells receive glutamatergic synapses from mossy fiber terminals and an inhibitory GABAergic input from the Golgi cell axons. Both amino-3-hydroxy-5-methyl-4-isoxazolepropionate (AMPA) and Nmethyl-D-aspartate (NMDA) receptors mediate excitatory signals from mossy fibers to the granule cells. Theta bursts of mossy fibre stimulation not only induce presynaptic long-term potentation (LTP) but also lead to enhanced intrinsic excitability of the granule cell [10].

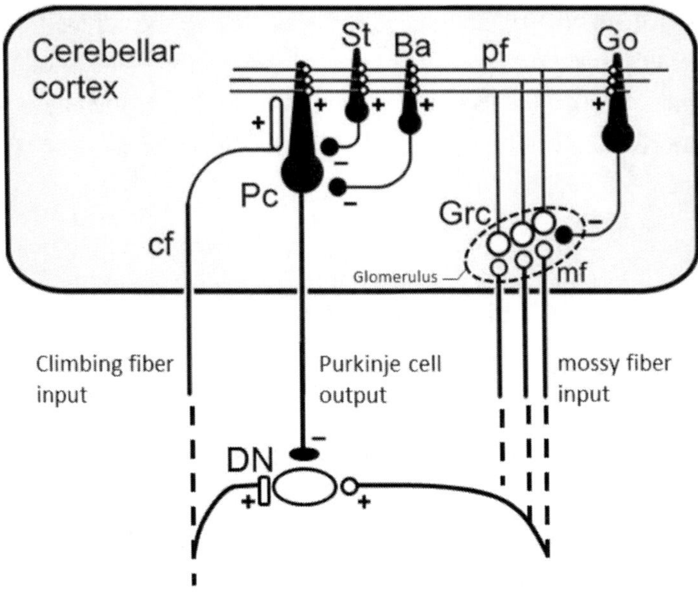

Figure 2. Schematic representation of cerebellar circuit. The cerebellar circuitry has two main afferent pathways. Mossy fibers (MF) from the brainstem and the spinal cord target the glomerulus at the granular layer and make synapses with granular cells (Gr). Within the glomerulus, the dendrites of Gr cells receive excitatory synapses from MF axon terminals and an inhibitory (-) input from the Golgi cell (G) axons. The axons of granule cells bifurcate into the parallel fibers (PF) in the molecular layer and supply glutamatergic synapses (+) to the dendritic tree of Purkinje cells (P). The PF make excitatory synapses not only with the distal dendrites of the Purkinje cells, but also those of inhibitory interneuron stellate (S) and basket cells (B). The other afferent pathway to the cerebellar cortex is the climbing fibers (CF) which arise from the inferior oliva and make several excitatory synapses with a single Purkinje neuron.

The enhanced excitability results from an increased input resistance and lowered spike threshold, which enhances excitatory postsynaptic potentials (EPSPs) and facilitates spike output. Further modification of spike output may be due to changes in intrinsic excitability resulting from NMDAR and gamma-aminobutryic acid (GABA) receptor activation in granule cells [10]. Thus, although granule cells have low background firing rates owing to tonic inhibition by Golgi cells, sensory activation can cause bursting in granule cells, such that mossy fibre input is transmitted with high reliability, yet in a modifiable manner, to Purkinje cells [11-13]. The axons of granule cells bifurcate into the parallel fibers in the molecular layer and supply glutamatergic synapses to the dendritic tree of Purkinje cells. Excitatory responses in the dendrites of Purkinje cells are mediated entirely by non-NMDA receptors. AMPA receptors generate fast EPSPs (excitatory postsynaptic potentials) and the glutamate metabotropic receptor mGluR1 is responsible for slow EPSPs [14]. The parallel fibers make excitatory synapses not only with the Purkinje cells, but also with two types of molecular layer interneurons, basket and Stella cells. Both are inhibitory interneurons and produce IPSPs currents in the Purkinje membrane with $GABA_A$ receptors [15].Climbing fibers are the other afferent pathway to the cerebellar cortex which arise from the inferior oliva. They make several excitatory synapses with Purkinje cells dendrites. Activation of the climbing fiber glutamatergic input powerfully excites cerebellar Purkinje cells via hundreds of widespread dendritic synapses, inducing a burst of known as complex spike. Following powerful complex spike activity, simple spikes can be suppressed [16].

The data reviewed above indicate that distributed plasticity in both the granule cell network and the Purkinje cell network support activity-dependent changes in synaptic efficacy [7]. Plasticity in the granule cell network may increase the diversity of coding, whereas plasticity in the Purkinje cell network may facilitate the selection of the appropriate coding and transfer it to the output domain that modulates the appropriate command. The combination of the different forms of plasticity in these networks during learning is refered as distributed synergistic plasticity: distributed because it includes various types of synaptic and intrinsic plastic effects in various types of neurons and superimposed interneurons in both the granular and molecular layer under compatible induction protocols; and synergistic because the different forms of long-term plasticity in the cerebellar cortex act synergistically [7]. Forms of plasticity that occur in serial manner (that is, plasticity in granule cell network and plasticity in Purkinje cell network) and forms of plasticity that occur in parallel manner (that is, plasticity at parallel fibre–Purkinje cell synapses and that at parallel fibre–interneuron synapses) in effect enhance one another through precise and periodic timing in the climbing fibre system relative to the mossy fibre system [7].

Long-term depression (LTD) has been proposed as the major memory mechanism in the cerebellum which is related to motor [17] and perceptual learning [18]. The coincidence of parallel fiber and climbing fiber activation induces LTD [19]. When the impulses of a group of parallel fibers and one climbing fiber reach the same Purkinje neuron synchronously and repeatedly, LTD will take place [17]. LTD will lead to a prolonged depression in postsynaptic sensitivity to glutamate [19]. The convergence of parallel and climbing fiber impulses on Purkinje cells also induces activity-dependent changes in molecular layer interneurons [20]. After pairing both inputs, the activation of these inhibitory interneurons will increase. Thus, two synergistic mechanisms contribute to long-term depression of Purkinje cells: LTD in Purkinje synapses and LTP in the parallel synapses with stellate and basket cells [15]. Postsynaptic LTP in Purkinje synapses can be reliably induced by lowfrequency parallel fibre stimulation without climbing fibre stimulation (Table 1). Induction of postsynaptic LTP requires a postsynaptic Ca^{2+} transient that is relatively small compared to that for LTD induction [7]. Postsynaptic LTP in parallel fiber- Purkinje synapses may have a homeostatic function. Once induced, it is able to remove and reset LTD after saturation, permitting in turn a new LTD [7].

Both types of molecular layer interneuron, that is, stellate cells and basket cells, are innervated by parallel fibres and able to induce LTD in the Purkinje synapses [7]. The activation of mGluR in parallel fiber-Purkinje synapses triggers the phospholipase C cascade linked to diaglicerol(DAG) and inositol trisphosphate (IP3) as second messengers. DAG activates protein kinase C (PKC) and IP3 generates Ca^{2+} release from intracellular stores. It has been also observed that nitric oxide (NO) and cyclic GMP cascade is part of the same molecular pathway [7].

Molecular events that trigger endocannabinoid-mediated short-term synaptic changes in the cerebellar cortex are shown to be both dependent and independent on Ca^{2+} current flowing into the postsynaptic cell. Activity-dependent long-term changes in the efficacy of cerebellar synapses are also mediated by an endocannabinoid-dependent retrograde mechanism [21, 22].

Table 1. Summary of all forms of long-term plasticity in cerebellar cortex

Cell type	Synapse	Main receptors	Long-term plasticity	Pre- or post-synaptic	Typical protocol	Key cascades
Granule cell (GrC)	MF-GrC	AMPA, NMDA	↑LTP, ↓LTD	Pre	MF burst, long	NMDAR, PKA
Golgi cell (GoC)	PF-GoC	AMPA, NMDA, kainate	↓LTD	Post	100Hz PF	PKA, mGluR2
Purkinje cell (PC)	PF-PC	AMPA	↑LTP	Pre	4 - 8 Hz PF	cAMP, PKA
			↓LTD	Pre	4 Hz PF	CB1R, NMDA
			↑LTP	Post	1 Hz PF	PP, NSF, NO
			↓LTD	Post	1 Hz PF + CF	PKC, PICK1, PKA, PKG, CaMKII, CRF, NMDAR, mGluR
	MLI-PC	$GABA_A$	↓LTD	NA	1 Hz MLI + CF	NA
	CF-PC	AMPA, NMDA	↑LTP, ↓LTD	Pre	5 Hz CF	Post Ca^{2+}
			↑LTP	Post	PC + CF	Post Ca^{2+}
			↓LTD	Post	5 Hz CF	mGluR, PKA, PKC, CRF
Molecular layer interneuron (MLI)	MLI-MLI	$GABA_A$	↑LTP	Pre	100 Hz PF	NMDAR, PKA
	PF-MLI	AMPA, NMDA	↑LTP	Pre	8 Hz PF	PKA, cAMP
			↓LTD	Pre	30 Hz PF	mGluR1, CB1R
			↑LTP, ↓LTD	Post	2 - 4 Hz PF	NO, mGluR, cAMP

CaMKII, Ca2+/calmodulin-dependent protein kinase II; cAMP, cyclic AMP; CB1R, cannabinoid 1 receptor; CF, climbing fibre; CRF, corticotropin releasing factor; $GABA_A$, GABA type A; $GABA_B$, GABA type B; LTD, long-term depression; LTP, long-term potentiation; MF, mossy fibre; mGLuR, metabotropic glutamate receptor; NA, not applicable; NMDAR, NMDA receptor; NO, nitric oxide; NSF, *N*-ethylmaleimide-sensitive factor; PICK1, protein-interacting with C kinase 1; PKA, cAMP-dependent protein kinase; PKC, protein kinase C; PKG, cyclic guanylate monophosphate-dependent protein kinase; PF, parallel fibre; PP, protein phosphatase; Arrows up or down indicate final effect on synaptic strength or excitability.

The repeated coincidence of parallel fiber and climbing fiber inputs triggers an enhancement of Ca^{2+} influx to the Purkinje neuron, mGluR postsynaptic activation and the endocannabinoid release to the synaptic cleft.

At the presynaptic site, plasticity at the parallel fibre–Purkinje cell synapse is dominated by potentiation and the control thereof by endocannabinoids. Presynaptic LTP, which is independent of postsynaptic activity, can be elicited by a relatively short period of activity in parallel fibres [7] (Table 1). This induces a presynaptic Ca^{2+}influx that activates a pathway involving Ca^{2+}/calmodulin-sensitive adenylyl cyclase, which in turn leads to a rise in cAMP and subsequent activation of cAMP-dependent PKA [7]. PKA activation may further increase the number and size of presynaptic Ca^{2+} transients, thereby probably further strengthening the potentiation. In addition, nitric oxide (NO) released from other synapses may contribute, through diffusion, to the induction of presynaptic LTP in non-activated parallel fibre terminals. This NO release might be initiated by activation of NMDARs at sites other than parallel fibres [7]. It is possible that a short-lasting form of presynaptic potentiation, which can be induced by a periodic burst pattern of homosynaptic stimulation of parallel fibres, can facilitate the initiation of presynaptic LTP at the parallel fibre–Purkinje cell synapse [7]. By contrast, activation of cannabinoid 1 (CB1) receptors following climbing fibreevoked release of endocannabinoids suppresses adenylyl cyclase 1, and thereby attenuates cAMP-dependent PKA activity and induction of presynaptic LTP.

4. Cerebellar Neuroplasticity Mechanisms Related to Addiction

Addiction includes a breakdown in motivational homeostasis, a disruption in reward processing and its modulation [25, 26]. Interestingly, prescription opioid-dependent patients have decreased functional connectivity at rest between reward structures and the cerebellum, including crus I [2]. In opioid-dependent patients, cerebellar functional connectivity with the nucleus accumbens and the amygdala decreased relative to age–

gender matched controls [2]. This change in functional correlation suggests that these reward regions are decoupled from cerebellar activation, indicating that opioid-dependent patients have disrupted communication between these regions.

Drug-induced long-term changes have been known as the substrate of addictive behavior [27, 28]. Thus, the compulsive phenotype of drug-seeking and drug-taking behavior, the relapse after withdrawal and the loss of control over drug use are all aspects of addictive behavior that result from the"re-wiring" of motivational circuitry after repeated exposure to drugs [24].

As illustrated in the previous section, short-term and long-term plasticity in the cerebellum seems to be mediated by glutamate and endocannabinoid-dependent cellular mechanisms. Additionally, it is known that the vermis of the cerebellum receives dopaminergic projections from the VTA [22]. As a result, it can be expected that drug-induced long-term neuroplasticity affects the interactions between glutamatergic inputs to the basal ganglia and the dopamine/endocannabinoid system.

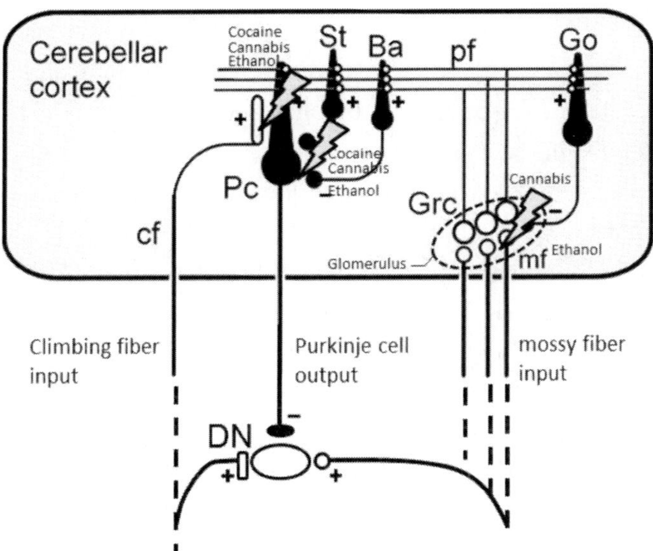

Figure 3. Drug potential action sites in the cerebellum. See Table 3 for further explanation.

4.1. The Neural Sites of Cerebellar Circuits Which are Affected by Addictive Drugs

4.1.1. Ethanol

Alcoholism is a debilitating disorder that can take a signifcant toll on health and professional and personal relationships [29]. Excessive alcohol consumption can have a serious impact on both drinkers and developing fetuses, leading to long-term learning impairments. Decades of research in laboratory animals and humans have demonstrated numerous molecular targets in cerebellar cortex where ethanol can act and stimulate or inhibit plasticity mechanisms (Figure 3). Acute alcohol consumption causes deficits in motor coordination and gait, suggesting an involvement of cerebellar circuits, which play a role in the fine adjustment of movements and in motor learning [29, 30]. It has previously been shown that ethanol modulates inhibitory transmission in the cerebellum and affects synaptic transmission and plasticity at excitatory climbing fiber (CF) to Purkinje cell synapses [3].

Cerebellar structural deficits have been frequently characterized clinically in alcoholism, with structural MRI studies and computed tomography studies in living patients [2], complementing findings from post-mortem studies [31]. In these studies, chronic alcoholism is linked to gray and white matter deficits in the anterior superior cerebellar vermis, although deficits in the inferior vermis and the cerebellar hemispheres have also been reported. A voxel-based morphometry (VBM) study found that patients with severe alcohol dependence showed significant gray matter deficits in crus II, along with white matter deficits in lobule VI [32]. These deficits were correlated with the neuropsychological measures of degraded executive function. Note that the deficits observed with chronic alcoholism in crus II and lobule VI, located in the posterior cerebellar hemispheres, have also been observed with cocaine and heroin use [2]. As a caveat, these structural changes may also be associated with vitamin B deficiency and other aspects of poor nutritional status [2]. Chronic intake of alcohol will increase the possibility of the cerebellum shrink. In the adult rat, these volumetric reductions may be due to death and atrophy of cells in the Purkinje, granular, and molecular layers of the cerebellar cortex [2]. In addition to degenerative changes in cell bodies, morphological changes to dendrites and axons have also been reported [22]. Combined treatments of thiamine defciency and alcohol exposure have led to axon terminal degeneration in the deep cerebellar nuclei, the sole output region for the cerebellum [3, 33]. Fewer synapses between parallel fibers and Purkinje cells [3] and a signifcant decrease in the number of dendritic microtubules have been found in alcohol-fed adult rats [3, 34]. Cerebellar structural abnormalities also appear in the developing cerebellum as a result of excessive early alcohol exposure. This damaging effect appears to be sensitive to time of alcohol exposure as rats receiving alcohol on postnatal day 4 suffered up to 50% Purkinje cell loss, whereas later exposure (postnatal days 8/9) resulted in less severe (15%) cell loss [3]. Alcohol-related damage in granule cells has also been investigated and cell vulnerability again appears to be greatest early in development (postnatal days 4/5) [3]. The structural integrity of the cerebellar deep nuclei, a region believed to be crucially important for EBC memory formation and storage [3], has been shown to be susceptible to chronic alcohol consumption.

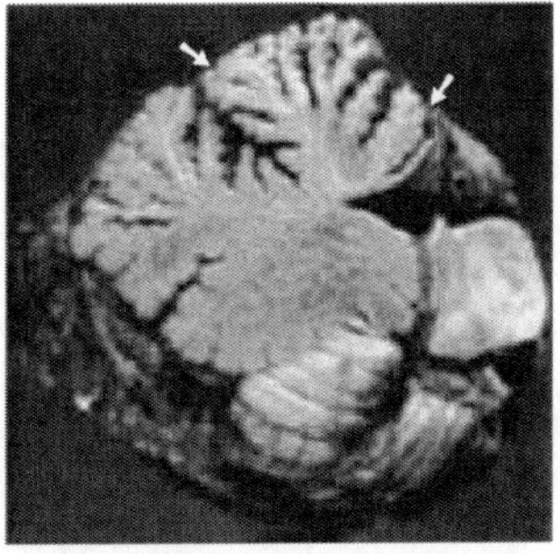

Figure 4. Pathological degeneration of the anteror cerebellum (arrows) caused by chronic alcohol abuse [50].

At the molecular and cellular level, Ethanol binds to the $GABA_A$ receptor to increase the inhibitory effects of the neurotransmitter GABA in the cerebellum. Ethanol is known to enhance -aminobutyric acid (GABA)–mediated transmission and to impair glutamatergic transmission [33]. Moreover, ethanol affects voltage-gated calcium channels [33]. It thus seems likely that ethanol can impair cerebellar function by interfering with synaptic transmission properties. It has indeed been shown that ethanol application depresses Purkinje cell activity and that this effect is partially mediated by an increase in GABAergic input [33].

Table 2. Effects of alcohol on cerebellar structure and function reported in the literature

Structural alterations	Ref.	Functional alterations	Ref.
Purkinje, granule and deep cerebellar nuclear cell loss	[51]	Greater inhibitory inputs to Purkinje cells	[44]
Dendritic microtubules loss	[52]	Slower increases in deep nuclear activity	[45]
Longer and reduced Purkirje dendritic spines	[53]	Purkinje cell firing differences	[46]
Increased climbing fbers	[54]	Greater cerebellar fMRI activation	[47]
Fewer synapses between parallel fbers and Purkinje cells	[3]	Greater fMRI responses in lobule VI	[3]
Cerebellar vermis gray matter defcits	[55]	More extensive cerebellar fMRI activation	[48]
Cerebellar peduncles damage	[56]	Greater crus I and vermis IV–V activation	[49]
Reductions in cerebellar cranial vault and volume	[57]		
Diminished white matter fiber	[58]		
Hypoplasia of cerebellar vermis	[59]		
Cerebellar volume loss	[60]		

A summary of animal and human work investigating how excessive alcohol consumption affects the cerebellum.

Ethanol also enhances GABAergic inhibition of granule cells, which has been attributed to increases in Golgi cell excitability and enhanced extrasynaptic $GABA_A$ receptor activity [33], respectively. The inhibitory effects of ethanol on glutamatergic transmission are most obvious for NMDA receptors [34, 35]. These receptors are expressed in Purkinje cells during development; only recently, functional NMDA receptors have been described at climbing fiber (CF) synapses onto mature Purkinje cells [36]. Ethanol indeed inhibits the late phase of CF-evoked complex spikes, but this downregulation is due to an inhibition of mGluR1 receptors, which can mediate slow, metabotropic currents (mGluR1 excitatory postsynaptic currents [EPSCs]) on CF activation [33]. Early complex spike components and CF–EPSCs remained unaffected by ethanol application [37], suggesting that ethanol does not modulate AMPA receptor function in Purkinje cells. Ethanol effects on parallel fiber (PF) synaptic transmission have not been reported.

In addition to modulating synaptic transmission through diverse pre- and postsynaptic mechanisms, ethanol has been shown to affect forms of synaptic plasticity and learning. Ethanol has been described to impair hippocampal long-term potentiation (LTP) and long-term depression (LTD) as well as striatal LTP [33]. In the cerebellum, LTD and LTP at PF synapses onto Purkinje cells are likely involved in forms of motor learning [38]. Impaired PF–LTD has been described in mice that were prenatally exposed to ethanol to mimic fetal alcohol syndrome [39]. Moreover, ethanol blocks the induction of CF–LTD [37], which could result in indirect consequences for PF synaptic plasticity because CF coactivation leads to PF–LTD induction, whereas PF stimulation alone induces PF–LTP [33]. Ethanol also influences cerebellar intracellular pathways associated with glutamate transmission [40]. By activating the intracellular signal transduction pathway of the serine/theorine kinase known as mitogen-activated protein kinase (MAPK) or extracellular signal regulated protein kinase (ERK), glutamate receptors control transcriptional activity and protein synthesis in response to drugs and thus, plasticity mechanisms leading to addiction [27]. Continuous regimen of ethanol treatment reduces the levels of ERK activation in the cerebellum, amygdala, hippocampus and cerebral cortex. On the contrary, intermittent exposure to ethanol up-regulates the MAPK-ERK pathway during withdrawal periods in the amygdala and cerebellum [41]. It has been shown that activations of the ERK pathway increase CREB-dependent transcription of an associated family of genes [27]. Moreover, CREB-mediated transcription is reported to be necessary for activating long-term plasticity genes [42]. In accordance, ethanol increases CREB levels in the cerebellum and this effect requires protein kinase A (PKA) and adenosine receptor activation (A2) [43]. Supporting the idea that ethanol produces cerebellar long-term plasticity, it has been recently demonstrated that ethanol affects dynamic modulation of the actin cytoskeketon in this structure [33]. Actin remodelling has been described as a crucial step for long-term memory storage in the hippocampus and other parts of the brain [33].

4.1.2. Cannabis Sativa

Cannabis sativa is an annual herbaceous flowering plant indigenous to eastern Asia but now of cosmopolitan distribution due to widespread cultivation [61]. The flowers (and to a lesser extent the leaves, stems, and seeds) of cannabis sativa contain psychoactive chemical compounds known as cannabinoids that are consumed for recreational, medicinal and spiritual purposes. Until now few studies have approached molecular or electrophysiological modifications induced by Cannabis sativa in the cerebellum (Figure 3). There are some reports show an increase in 2-AG (2-arachidonoylglycerol) in the cerebellum of chronic Δ9-tetrahydro-cannnabinol-treated rats as compared with controls [22]. Δ9- tetrahydro-cannabinol (Delta-9-THC) is the major psychoactive component of cannabis sativa and primary ingredient in marijuana. Chronic delta-9-THC administration prevents the increase in the ERK pathway produce by acute delta-9-THC administration [61]. However, after withdrawal an up-regulation of adenylcyclase activity [22] and a downstream enhancement of the cAMP-PKA pathway [22] are both observed. Changes in CREB expression can be seen in granule cells at granular layer of the cerebellum after delta-9-THC treatment. Acute delta-9-THC increased CREB immunostaining and protein expression, although a significant decrease in CREB was observed in chronically treated rats. The decrease still persisted 3 weeks after withdrawal [62].

The cerebellum contains the cannabinoid receptors CB1 and CB2, inhibitory G-protein coupled receptors that bind to cannabinoids. Additional data demonstrated that the endocannabinoid system mediates plasticity changes induced by other drugs of abuse in the cerebellum. For example, the endocannabinoid system seems to be involved in molecular mechanisms of ethanol and morphine. Chronic ethanol or morphine exposure to cultures of cerebellar granule cells produces accumulation of 2-arachidonylglycerol and arachidonylethanolamide (AEA) [63-65]. The synthesis of these endocannabinoids increases proportionally to the duration of the ethanol exposure and is prevented by CB1 antagonist [64]. Also, the density of CB1 receptors could be reduced by both drugs in the cerebellum, but a recovery at the basal levels is observed after 24 hours of withdrawal from ethanol [64, 65].

In spite of the above potential effects, a consistent pattern of cerebellar changes with marijuana (cannabis) usage has not been apparent across structural studies [2], nor across resting state metabolism studies using positron emission tomography (PET) [2]. When cerebellar structural changes are detected, they appear as increases in the anterior cerebellum [66] and the inferior posterior vermis [2], decreases in white matter volume [2]. Some evidence suggests that the posterior cerebellum has lower resting cerebral blood flow in marijuana users after monitored abstinence versus controls [2].

4.1.3. Cocaine

Cocaine is a crystalline tropane alkaloid derived from the coca plant, and acts as a serotoninnorepinephrine-dopamine reuptake inhibitor. Both serotonin receptors and norepinephrine receptors are expressed in the cerebellum. A VBM study on cocaine use and brain structure [67] suggests that drug use impacts specific regions within the cerebellum. This study compared gray and white matter in 40 cocaine abusers and 41 matched healthy controls, and found that abusers had significantly reduced gray matter in Lobule VI, Crus I, and Crus II. The finding of reduced gray matter in Lobule VI in cocaine abusers was also corroborated recently in another VBM study [68]. Lobule VI, Crus I, and Crus II are located in the posterior cerebellar hemispheres, which have been related to modulation of affect and cognition in clinical studies on cerebellar stroke [69].

Despite the fact that several data have supportedthe involvement of the cerebellum in the functional alterations observed after prolonged cocaine use, this brain structure has been traditionally ignored and excluded from the circuitry affected by addictive drugs.

Cocaine-dependent neuronal plasticity includes molecular and structural modifications in the cortical–striatal–limbic networks with a ventral to dorsal gradient [2]. In addition, cocaine induce restrictive metaplasticity in such a way so that the probability of any new change is decreased [70].

Increasing evidence has demonstrated that cocaine induced a large increase in cerebellar proBDNF levels and its expression in Purkinje neurons, with the mature BDNF expression remaining unchanged. Together with this, cocaine-treated mice exhibited a substantial enhancement of D3 receptor levels. Both ΔFosB and AMPA receptor Glu2 subunit expressions were enhanced in cocaine-treated animals. Significant pruning in Purkinje dendrite arborization and reduction in the size and density of Purkinje boutons contacting deep cerebellar projection neurons accompanied cocaine-dependent increase in proBDNF. Cocaine-associated effects point to the inhibitory Purkinje function impairment, as was evidenced by lower activity in these cells. Moreover, the probability of any remodelling in Purkinje synapses appears to be decreased due to an upregulation of extracellular matrix components in the PNNs surrounding the medial nuclear neurons. cocaine is also able to promote plasticity modifications in the cerebellum of sensitized animals similar to those in the basal ganglia [70, 71].

4.1.4. Nicotine

Nicotine is a parasympathomimetic alkaloid, which acts as a nicotinic acetylcholine receptor agonist. In the cerebellum, these receptors control the release of the neurotransmitters glutamate, GABA, and norepinephrine. VBM studies in cigarette smokers vs. healthy controls have demonstrated reduced gray matter in the posterior cerebellar hemispheres, specifically in Lobule VI and Crus I [2]. Gray matter volume in Crus I was also found to be correlated negatively to the magnitude of nicotine dependence [2]. The effect of nicotine on cerebellar structure has recently been reviewed in detail [2].

4.1.5. Opioids

Because of their potent analgesic properties, opiate drugs have been used for centuries. Opiates include compounds derived from the opium poppy such as morphine and codeine, as well as many synthetic derivatives such as heroin, oxycodone, and hydrocodone.

Opioids such as heroin act on opioid receptors in the brain, of which mu and kappa varieties are present in the human cerebellum [72]. Regarding the impact of opiates on structure, the volume of cerebellar cortex is significantly reduced in children who were exposed to heroin in utero [73]. In this study, gray matter differences were evaluated in 14 exposed versus 14 control children using a region of interest analysis. When accounting for age, gestational age and gender, cerebellar white matter and cerebellar cortex showed a significant loss in gray matter, along with the accumbens, putamen, pallidum, amygdala and cerebral cortex overall. Although these structural changes were reported as the main findings, the only significant effect was in the cerebellar cortex when intracranial volume was included as a factor. Considering that intracranial volume is highly variable in children of different ages, this serves to highlight the vulnerability of the cerebellum to heroin exposure during prenatal development.

A recent DTI study in ex-heroin users reported a reduction in mean fractional anisotropy (FA) in the cerebellum [74]. Using DTI, 30 ex-heroin users on either methadone or buprenorphine maintenance medication were compared with 29 age–gender matched healthy controls. Bora et al. found lower FA, degraded white matter integrity, in the superior and middle cerebellar peduncles. These cerebellar peduncles serve as major pathways for afferent and efferent neural information flow between the cerebellum and the midbrain, including the pons. The implication that these white matter tracts are degraded with a history of heroin abuse suggests that addiction is related to a disruption in cerebellar processing and connectivity with other brain regions.

There are many reports of synaptic plasticity induced by acute opiates. As with cocaine and other abused drugs, a single injection of morphine was found to increase the ratio of AMPA to NMDA excitatory postsynaptic currents 24 hours after administration, consistent with LTP of glutamatergic synapses onto dopamine neurons [75]. Recently, it has also been reported that acute morphine induces AMPAR receptor redistribution in a manner similar to cocaine, specifically an insertion of GluA2-lacking AMPARs

[76]. These data are consistent with earlier work that GluA1, but not GluA2, overexpression sensitizes animals to morphine's locomotor-activating and rewarding behaviors [22]. Acute opiates also influence plasticity at GABAergic synapses. High-frequency stimulation has been found to elicit LTP at GABA terminals (LTP_{GABA}), an effect that is dependent on activation of postsynaptic NMDA receptors and release of NO as a retrograde messenger [77]. NO then increases guanylyl cyclase (GC) activity in the GABA neuron, leading to increased GABA release and LTP_{GABA}. A single dose of morphine inhibits LTP_{GABA} by interrupting the NO–GC–protein kinase G (PKG) signal cascade, causing a loss of normal inhibitory control (observed 2 and 24 hours following injection, but not 5 days) [77, 78]. Thus, disruption of LTP_{GABA} provides another mechanism for the ability of acute opiates to increase dopamine neuronal activity.

4.1.6. Psychostimulants

Although the cerebellum has relatively low dopamine innervation, it is known that VTA sends dopamine (DA) projections to the vermis [79]. In accordance, dopamine transporters and axons labelled for tyrosine hydroxilase have been found in the vermis [80]. As should be expected, cocaine and amphetamine increase Fos-like immunoreactivity in the rat granular layer of the vermis at a wide range of doses and, occasionally in Purkinje neurons [81] (Figure 3). Recordings of extracellular activity in the cerebelar cortex showed that cocaine is able to suppress spontaneous firing and glutamate-induced activation of Purkinje cells [22]. It would appear that cocaine-induced inhibition of these cells is mediated by a DA-independent mechanism. Both spontaneous firing and glutamate-dependent suppression are blocked with yohimbine, an 2-adrenoreceptor antagonist [22]. Thus, it is very likely that the mechanism underlying the effect of cocaine on Purkinje neurons is the inhibition of noradrenaline transporters at synapses neuromodulated by noradrenergic fibers from the locus coeruleus [22].

One of the neuroadaptations that has been recently confirmed in the Purkinje soma and dendrites after cocaine administration is the augmented expression of Homer 1b/c and 3a/b [104]. These long homer isoforms are a crucial link between mGluR and IP3-dependent intracellular Ca^{2+} signalling, and they are considered as an important step of synaptic remodelling and spine morphogenesis [22].

In conclusion, the cellular and molecular actions of addictive drugs in the cerebellum involve long-term adaptative changes in receptors, neurotransmitters and intracellular signalling transduction pathways that may lead to the "re-wiring" of cerebellar microzones and in turn change functional networks where the cerebellum is involved (Table 3). Several of the above-mentioned drug-induced molecular changes have been correlated with drug dependence, drug tolerance and the withdrawal syndrome [22]. In general, acute drug administration increases receptors, neurotransmitters and intracellular signalling transduction responses in the cerebellum. Compensatory changes during chronic treatment lead to an apparent normalization of these initial modifications, but after drug withdrawal alterations in cerebellar parameters can be seen again. It is important to note that intermittent drug administration can exacerbate plasticity changes observed during wash-out periods.

Homeostatic adaptations that may occur within cells and circuits after repeated stimulation by addictive drugs may increase the risk of relapse even after drug withdrawal. Thus, the new point of view about addiction involves both a compulsive pattern of drug consumption and the high risk of relapse as major symptoms of the addiction illness. This current view proposes that the compulsive phenotype of drug-seeking and drug-taking behavior and relapse are both aspects of addictive behavior that result from drug-induced long-term changes which re-wire motivational circuitry [24, 27, 28]. Neuroadaptations as sensitization and associative memory mechanisms are now considered crucial processes to explain addiction.

5. Drug-Induced Sensitization and Cerebellar Plasticity

Repeated exposure to drugs of abuse enhances the motor-stimulant response to these drugs, a phenomenon termed behavioral sensitization.

Animals that are extinguished from self-administration training readily relapse to drug, conditioned cue, or stress priming. The involvement of sensitization in reinstated drug-seeking behavior remains controversial. It is known that drug-induced modifications of the interactions between dopamine and glutamate systems, including changes in the structure and function of receptors and associated intracellular pathways, trigger a cascade of neuroadaptations underlying acquired increases in sensitivity to the behavioral effects of addictive drugs [24, 82, 83].

The relevance of sensitization for the development of addiction has been suggested by the theory of Incentive Salience [83, 84]. It proposes that as a consequence of long-term changes in the dopaminergic system the incentivemotivational ability of drug-associated cues is sensitized and contributes to intensify drug craving and drug seeking. Sensitization could also reinforce associations between conditioned cues and drug effects leading to the strength of conditioned memories, which in turn could trigger drug seeking and drug taking [85, 86]. The simplest way to asses if an animal sensitized is testing its locomotor activity during repeated administration of the drug. The progressive increase in locomotor activity and the significant difference between the first and the last day of drug treatment show the sensitization of the drug effect. Locomotor sensitization is a common and robust behavioral alteration in rodents whereby following exposure to abused drugs such as cocaine, the animal becomes significantly more hyperactive in response to an acute drug challenge.

Still few but consistent data demonstrate that the cerebellar cortex plays a key role in the neuroadaptations leading to behavioral sensitization. The cerebellum is a central site for the molecular mechanisms of 9-delta-THC sensitization [22]. 9-delta-THC sensitized rats show an increase in CB1 receptor binding restricted to the cerebellar cortex, with no appreciable alteration in other brain areas that also have a high density of CB1 receptors [22]. Since previous reports revealed that CB1 down-regulation correlates with the development of 9-delta-THC tolerance [87], the increase in the binding seems to be a specific adaptation underlying sensitization.

Table 3. Drug Molecular Mechanisms in the Cerebellum [22]

	Affected function	Acute	Chronic	Under Withdrawal
Ethanol	• Glutamate function • GABA function • CB1 function • Intracelullar pathways and associated gene expression	• Depression of Ca2+ signalling linked to AMPAR in Purkinje neurons (30 - 100mM) • Enhancement in Ca2+ current to mGLuR agonists in Purkinje neurons (10mM) • Increase in GABAergic inhibition of granule cell via excitation of Golgi cells • Increase in GABA-mediated inhibitory responses of Purkinje neurons • Nicotine enhances ethanol-induced depression of Purkinje neurons • Loss of F-actin	• Increase in Ca2+ signaling linked to AMPAR in Purkinje neurons • Reduction in responsiveness to externally applied GABA in granule cells • Accumulation of endocannabinoids • Reduction in CB1 density • Down-regulation of ERK activation • Induction of cAMP-dependent gene expression regulated by CREB and PKA	• Up-regulation of ERK activation
Delta-9-THC	• Intracelullar pathways and associated gene expression	• Up-regulation of ERK activation • Increase in CREB expression	• Down-regulation ERK activation • Decrease in CREB expression	• Up-regulation of adenycyclase activity • Up-regulation of the cAMPPKA pathway • Decrease in CREB expression
Psychostimulants	• Glutamate function • Intracellular pathways and associated gene expression	• Suppression of spontaneous firing and glutamate-induced activation of Purkinje cells • Adrenergic agonist increases cocaine dependent suppression of Purkinje neurons	• Increase in FOS expression at the granular layer • Increase in Homer 1b/c and 3a/b expression in Purkinje neurons	

Repeated and intermittent exposure of ethanol sensitizes locomotion [88]. It has been shown that the intermittent regimen of ethanol treatment activates phosphorylated ERK that peaks 24 hours post-withdrawal in the rat cerebellum and amygdala [22]. In another study, the possibility of alcohol-induced sensitivity to gluten was investigated. The presence of TG2 antibodies (the autoantigen of celiac disease) in patients with chronic alcoholism raised the possibility of alcohol induced sensitivity. Alcohol related cerebellar degeneration may, in genetically susceptible individuals, induce sensitization to gluten. Such sensitization may result from a primary cerebellar insult, but a more systemic effect is also possible [22].

Sensitization to cocaine has been also associated with several cerebellar molecular changes. Chronic administration of cocaine that induces locomotor sensitization also increases the binding of MK-801, a NMDA antagonist, in the cerebellum [89]. Finally, sensitization of c-fos and jun-B mRNA has been demonstrated in the cerebellar cortex of cocaine sensitized rats [90]. This effect is mediated by D1, D2, GABAB and NMDA cerebellar receptors.

Further research is required to elucidate if the involvement of the cerebellum in drug-induced sensitization is general for all drug-induced sensitized effects, or rather, if it is restricted to locomotion, since lobules IX and X are directly involved in the control of locomotor functions [91].

5.1. Cerebellar Role in Drug Craving

A cerebellar role in drug craving has been demonstrated with cues for heroin [92, 94], cocaine [23, 95] and alcohol [93]. Cerebellar activity has been correlated with self-reports of 'feeling tense' and 'withdrawal symptoms' during cue evoked craving in heroin users [94]. Craving is particularly acute in heroin users, and evidence suggests that cerebellum has a role in opioid craving. A PET study in 10 male active heroin users measured rCBF responses to drug related and neutral video cues presented in separate scans [94]. After each scan, subjective ratings were collected on a scale of 1–10 for a variety of sensations, including withdrawal symptoms and feeling tense. Across both drug and neutral video cues, cerebellar blood flow was correlated with self-reports of severity of withdrawal symptoms and feeling tense. These findings suggest that cerebellar activation may reflect aversive sensations that are not specific to drug craving per se.

A recent fMRI study compared responses to drug image cues in short-term versus longterm abstinence in 19 male heroin users [92]. Greater cerebellar activation was found to heroin versus neutral cues with short-term abstinence, yet cerebellar deactivation was observed with long-term abstinence. The authors suggested that this meant that longterm abstinence decreased the salience of conditioned cues, with the cerebellar activation presumably reflecting stimulus salience. Also, an fMRI study found posterior cerebellar BOLD responses in abstinent alcoholics while presented with ethanol odors to induce craving [93].

An rCBF PET study that induced craving for cocaine also found a response in the left posterior cerebellar hemisphere [95]. Aside from the posterior hemispheres, the cerebellar vermis has also been found to respond to cues related to cocaine [23], methylphenidate [96] and alcohol [93] in cocaine-dependent subjects and alcoholics.

Converging evidence from structural and functional neuroimaging studies across a variety of drug conditions indicates that the cerebellar posterior hemispheres are significantly different in addicted subjects versus healthy controls. Yet to be determined is whether these differences in the cerebellum promote the development addiction or are simply a reflection of the pharmacological effects of drug use.

6. Addiction and Conditioned Emotional Memories in the Cerebellum

Emotion can have a powerful effect on humans and animals. Numerous studies have shown that the most vivid autobiographical memories tend to be of emotional events, which are likely to be recalled more often and with more clarity and detail than neutral events. The activity of emotionally enhanced memory retention can be linked to human evolution; during early development, responsive behavior to environmental events would have progressed as a process of trial and error. Survival depended on behavioral patterns that were repeated or reinforced through life and death situations. Through evolution, this process of learning became genetically embedded in humans and all animal species in what is known as flight or fight instinct.

The anatomical connections of the cerebellum with regions involved in emotion regulation and in perception of socially salient emotional material are revealing. The cerebellum is bidirectionally linked with regions subserving perception of socially salient material, including the posterior parietal cortex and pre-frontal regions [97, 98]. The cerebellum is particularly well-suited to regulate emotion, as connections with limbic regions, including the amygdala, the hippocampus, and the septal nuclei have been posited [99, 100]. In addition, reciprocal connections link the cerebellum with brainstem areas containing neurotransmitters involved in mood regulation, including serotonin, norepinepherine, and dopamine [101].

Two lines of research have shown cerebellum/emotion associations in humans: lesion studies and functional neuroimaging studies. Lesions of the posterior lobe and vermis of the cerebellum are associated with blunted affect as well as impairment in a variety of cognitive domains including those of executive function, spatial cognition, and language [69]. Functional neuroimaging studies designed to visually induce emotion [102] or requiring the recognition on an emotion in the face have found increases in cerebellar activity. A study that examined the neural correlates of perceived humor found a positive correlation between ratings of humor and cerebellar activity [103]. Damage to the posterior lobule of the cerebellum can lead to clinical cerebellar cognitive-affective syndrome (CCAS). Patients with CCAS may display affective symptoms, including changes in affect and emotional lability, without a cerebellar motor syndrome [104]. The affective disturbances in CCAS, which range from emotional blunting and depression to disinhibition and psychotic features, suggest that the posterior lobule of the cerebellum is involved in cognitive functioning and emotion. Several human neuroimaging studies involve the cerebellum, specially the vermis, in the reactivation of drugconditioned emotional memories [93, 96, 105,

106]. Neuroimaging studies show increased glucose metabolism elicited by cocaine-and ethanol-conditioned cues in the cerebellum [93, 96, 105, 106]. Grant et al. (1996) demonstrated that the paraphernalia associated with cocaine taking increased activation of the dorsolateral prefrontal cortex, the amygdala, and the cerebellum [105]. Interestingly, this pattern of activation was not observed for neutral videotapes. Later, they showed that when cocaine addicts listened to an evocative script that described in detail physiological and psychological sensations associated with cocaine use, the right cerebellum was also activated [106]. Cocaine- associated cues elicit greater increases in activation of lobules II, III, VIII, and IX [23]. Olfactory stimulation with ethanol in alcoholic patients under detoxification, but not in normal healthy controls, activates the right amygdala, hippocampus, insula and cerebellum [93].

Moreover, in another study, therapeutic intervention in alcoholic patients reduced subjective craving, accompanied by reductions in the cerebellar activity [93]. Therapeutic training, hence, seems to reorganize emotional memory networks where the cerebellum is a crucial node, or at least, is able to produce transient extinction-like effect in this network. Expectations are a central cognitive process in reward induced behavior [96]. The expectation of the drug effect is shown to modulate drug-associated responses in animal models of drug consumption [107, 108]. For example, dopaminergic activations are larger when animals are treated with cocaine in an environment where they previously received cocaine as opposed to a novel environment [107]. Also, cocaine induces greater dopamine release when it is self-administered compared to yoked administration [108]. In accordance, Volkow et al. (2003) [96] observed larger increases in cerebellum and thalamus glucose metabolism when cocaine addicts expected to receive drug and received it as compared with when they expected placebo and received drug. Conscious memory retrieval provoked by a cocaine themed interview correlates with larger activation in the cerebellum, amygdala, orbitofrontal, cortex, and insular cortex as compared with a neutral themed interview [22]. Taken together, human studies on drug-conditioned memories involve the cerebellum in both explicit and implicit memory. These are in accordance with other studies that demonstrate a cerebellar role in the consolidation of emotional aversive memory in rodents [22]; cognitive procedural learning consolidation [109] or episodic memory encoding in humans [110].

The recall and consolidation of conditioned emotional memories that are reactivated in an automatic or implicit mode, seems to be controlled, in part, by the vermis [22]. During cognitive procedural learning it has been observed that different regions of the cerebellum are activated depending on the phase of the learning. The vermis is only activated in the automatic phase [109]. The vermis connects to dopamine neurons in the VTA and substancia nigra [111] and the VTA sends dopaminergic projections to the vermis [111, 112], forming a reciprocal midbrain to cerebellar circuit. As a result of its connections, therefore, the vermis seems to be part of the circuit that sustains emotional memory and emotional behavior. Since there is almost no causal study to investigate the role of the cerebellum in conditioned memory, further animal research is crucial to implicate the cerebellum in the emotional memory circuitry.

7. Cerebellar Mechanisms Related to Motivated Behavior

Motivation and emotion embody features of a common core phenomenon, the motivational-emotional system, that interacts with general-purpose processing systems of conditioning, learning, higher order cognition and action [113]. Motivation can be defined as the internal drive of an organism, while emotions can be considered as the readout of this internal drive when activated by perceiving a challenging stimulus [113]. Emotions include a way of feeling and a way of acting [114]. Importantly, processes associated with motivation and emotion can be considered as phenomena that arise from disturbances in internal homeostasis of the body (e.g., hunger). The organism will initiate the proper action (e.g., eating) to restore internal homeostasis. From this viewpoint, motivation and emotion are not merely linked to goal-directed action [115]; they in fact constitute the origins of all human behavior.

Moreover, an important additional component is the ability of the organism to plan a behavioral strategy and to monitor the consequence of actions which allows the organism to fine-tune or regulate its behavior if the desired end state (e.g., homeostasis) is not yet reached. Affect is frequently used as a general term to describe processes related to motivation, emotion, and regulation. As such, action can be viewed as the physical expression of the organism's state of intentionality, which involves the integration of sensory and motor processes, execution of motor commands, monitoring, and modification. All of the above perfectly match the traditional functional descriptions of the cerebellum providing a theoretical argument favoring cerebellar contributions to motivation and emotion. The organizational properties of the cerebellum and its interconnections provide a neuroanatomical basis for a role of the cerebellum in motivation, emotion, and associated regulatory processes.

Addicts show an uncontrollable drive to seek drugs and show a decreased incentive to seek non-drug rewards. As a consequence of repeated use of addictive drugs, brain systems controlling motivated behavior are re-organized in a way that competes with plasticity induced by natural rewards, reducing the probability of natural rewards to activate goal-directed actions [22]. Goal-directed behavior is tuned by instrumental or reinforced learning so behavior can adapt to environmental and internal demands. By repeated experience, reinforcers increase the probability of the response that lead to seeking them. Instrumental learning, then, by selecting responses that allow access to the reinforcer produces an adaptive reduction in the behavioral repertory and initiates the transition fromm behavior controlled by their consequences to stimulus driven habits. Acquisition, storage, reactivation even reconsolidation of instrumental memories all involve a cross-talk between the prefrontal cortex and basal ganglia [85]. Three functional networks have been recognized to control the transition from goaldirected behavior to habit: the limbic network, the associative network and the sensorimotor network [22]. The limbic network is involved in the process of instrumental learning that is, learned behavior controlled by their consequences or goal-directed behavior. However, habit formation requires a shift of the activation from the prefrontal cortex-dorsomedial striatum circuit (associative network) to sensorimotor cortices-dorsolateral striatum circuit (sensorimotor network).

Motivational impact of drug-associated stimulus is strengthened leading to the transition from instrumental memories to inflexible drug-seeking habit formation. The progression from a ventral to a dorsolateral stream may be facilitated by dopamine signalling. Thus, as dopamine neuron activity sensitizes the transition from a goaldirected drug-induced behavior to compulsive drug-seeking is expected to be favored [85].

Human and animal studies have emphasized the importance of the prefrontal cortex for behavioral flexibility. For example, there are similarities between patients with prefrontal lesions and drug addicts [116, 117]. Both display an inflexible behavior and frequently are not aware of the risk of incurring future negative outcomes [117]. In addition, human addicts show a reduction in the prefrontal activation when they are tested during abstinence periods, but also show a hyperresponsiveness of the prefrontal cortex when they are challenged with the drug [118]. Finally, animal studies demonstrate that lesions of the prefrontal cortex impair extinction of drug consumption [116]. The same result is observed if the lesion is restricted to the mesocortical dopaminergic system [116], which has been proposed as being the system which signals when the goal representation should be updated to activate a new response [119].

8. Hypotheses Related to Addiction in the Cerebellum

In this section, we introduce two conceptual models of the role of cerebellum in addictive processes.

8.1. Impaired Response Inhibition and Salience Attribution

Given the supporting evidence, the cerebellum's role as a modulator can be readily adapted to existing models of addiction. In the context of neuroimaging, a major conceptual model for addiction is the impaired response inhibition and salience attribution (i-RISA) model [120], also described as a four-circuit model [96]. Briefly, the model consists of four interconnected circuits relating to memory, reward/saliency, executive control and motivation/drive. The response to a reward is mediated by the interactions of these four components. In the addicted brain, the homeostatic balance is drastically altered, such that the components for memory, reward/saliency and motivation/drive are amplified, and cognitive control is diminished. Different brain regions have been assigned to each circuit, such as the dorsolateral prefrontal cortex for control and the nucleus accumbens for reward. With the cerebellum's postulated function as a multimodal modulator of cognition, affect and aversion, the cerebellum is optimally configured to regulate brain processes directly involved in addiction (Figure 5). This cerebellar model for addiction proposes that the cerebellum plays an influential role in maintaining the homeostatic balance of the four circuits. In the addicted brain, structural gray matter deficits in lobule VI, lobule VIIb, crus I and crus II, and the vermis implicate changes in the cerebellum's ability to interact and communicate with brain regions related to the four circuits. These brain regions receive inputs from the deep cerebellar nuclei, the main output channels of the cerebellum. From the cerebellar cortex, the dentate and fastigial nuclei receive inputs from the lateral hemisphere and vermis, respectively. Within the dentate nuclei, separate cerebellar output channels have been identified that project to areas related to cognitive, skeletomotor (motor and premotor cortices) and oculomotor function (frontal eye fields) [2]. The fastigial nuclei have an output channel that relates to limbic processing, with projections to the hippocampus, amygdala and the cingulate cortex [121].

In addiction, decreased inhibition of brain regions, such as the hypothalamus, subgenual anterior cingulate and parahippocampal gyrus, would result in a net excitatory effect in brain circuits related to reward/salience, motivational drive and memory, as well as stress and interoception. Likewise, the reciprocal pathways between brain circuits related to executive control would be disrupted, interfering with the ability of the prefrontal cortex to inhibit unwanted drug seeking behavior.

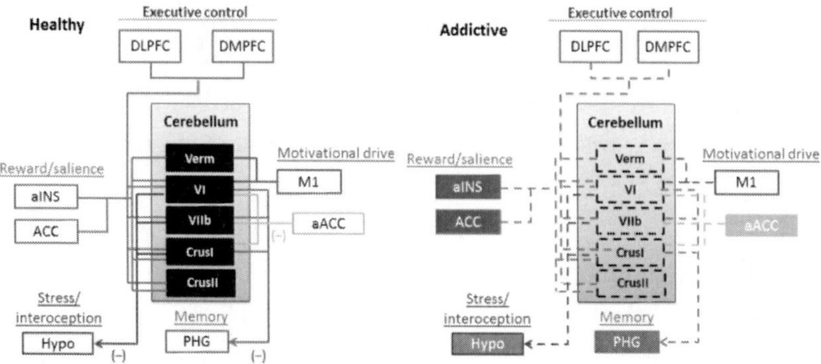

Figure 5. Impaired response inhibition and salience attribution cerebellar model for addiction. The right panel highlights the cerebellum's role as a modulator of affective and cognitive function in the healthy brain. This schematic highlights the four major brain networks proposed to be affected by addiction (adapted from [2]). The arrows show the proposed direction of cerebellar down modulation of specific brain regions within each circuit. The left panel proposes how cerebellar dysfunction may impact the addicted brain. The black dashed boxes highlight structural degradation of specifically localized cerebellar structures with addiction. The dashed lines show disrupted functional connectivity and cerebellar modulation of specific brain regions related to executive control, reward/salience, motivational drive and memory. The filled colored boxes and bold type represent brain circuits released from cerebellar modulation, leading to an uninhibited and sensitized neurological state. Note that all cerebellar outputs project through the deep cerebellar nuclei (refer to text for details). ACC = anterior cingulate cortex; aINS = anterior insula; DLPFC = dorsolateral prefrontal cortex; DMPFC = dorsomedial prefrontal cortex; Hypo = hypothalamus; M1 = primary motor cortex; PHG = parahippocampal gyrus; sACC = subgenual anterior cingulate cortex; Verm = vermis; VI = cerebellar hemispheric lobule VI; VIIb = cerebellar hemispheric lobule VIIb.

8.2. Drug-Induced Fronto-Cerebellar Network Reorganization

As reviewed in previous section, the cerebellum has reciprocal connections to functional circuitry responsible for motivated behavior. Fronto-cerebellar circuits deserve special consideration in the present case because it involves the cerebellum in the system for the executive control of voluntary behavior. Nonhuman primate studies have shown two dissociated fronto-cerebellar contralateral circuits: one circuit presents reciprocal connections between motor cortices and cerebellum, and the other has prefrontal-cerebellum reciprocal projections [122].

Ito has proposed that the prefrontal cortex and cerebellum work in parallel [123]. As a consequence of cerebellar plasticity, an internal model of prefrontal representation is created in the cerebellum. This internal model is a copy of the information stored in the prefrontal cortex. Thus, the cerebellum may act in parallel to the prefrontal cortex and be recruited when automatic processing and activation of voluntary behavior is required. Hence, it may be expected that the cerebellum is crucial to consolidate and perform automatic goal-directed behavior, and to contribute to the transition from instrumental behavior to habits.

Hester and Garavan (2003) studied GO-NOGO response inhibition tasks in cocaine users and detected worse perseverance inhibition in this group than in control subjects. As working memory demands increased, cocaine users showed non-responsiveness of anterior cingulate cortex accompanied by over responsiveness of the left cerebellum [124]. Cerebellar activation correlates inversely with performance. Nonetheless, an inverse pattern was seen in normal subjects. As demands increase, control subjects have over-activated cingulate cortices and prefrontal regions but cerebellar activation remains neutral [124]. In alcoholics, a similar pattern has been observed, but in this case the over-activity was detected in the right cerebellum [125].

Research into executive control in marijuana abusers strongly support the participation of the cerebellum in the executive function affected by drugs [126]. In the Iowa Gambling Task, marijuana abusers perform as prefrontal lesioned patients, drug addicts and pathological gamblers do [126]. All groups are hypersensitive to immediate rewards (disadvantage cards) and less sensitive to losses. Moreover, they learn from their previous mistakes slowly. Interestingly, this characteristic behavior was correlated with a specific brain activation pattern, which resembles findings of studies with cocaine users and alcoholics: less activation in the orbitofrontal and dorsomedial cortices along with greater activation in the cerebellum. Smokers and non-smokers also show differences in the pattern of brain activation when they are involved in a reward task [127]. The most apparent characteristic of smokers is an increase in the activity of the cerebellum during monetary and nonmonetary reward which contrasts with a wider pattern of activation in non-smokers, including striatum, and prefrontal and limbic cortices.

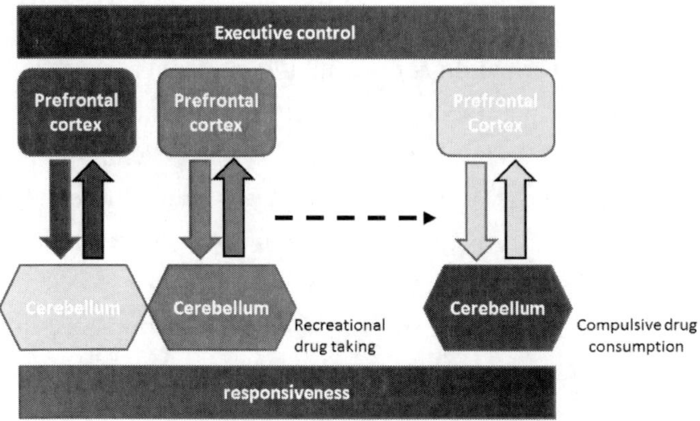

Figure 6. Drug-induced fronto-cerebellar network reorganization model. Functional and structural modifications induced by drugs in the cerebellum may enhance the susceptibility of fronto-cerebellar circuitry to be changed by repeated drug exposure. Drug-induced cerebellar hyper-responsiveness can cause a functional reorganization of the fronto-cerebellar network and reduce the executive control of the prefrontal cortex on behavior. One can expect the pattern of cerebellar hyperactivity and prefrontal hypoactivity to follow a temporal gradient, the cerebellum being more important as the exposure to drugs is repeated. The top and bottom bars show a white (minimum)-dark (maximum) gradient to express changes in the executive control of the prefrontal cortex (top) and responsiveness (bottom).

Altogether, the above-discussed results suggest that prefrontal and cerebellar nodes in the prefrontal-cerebellar loop are recruited in a competitive manner. In non-pathological individuals, when cognitive demands are high prefrontal executive control is activated. When an automatic and rapid response is required, however, the cerebellum increases its activity and prefrontal cortex activity reduces its activation. Indeed, in addict subjects, prefrontal-cerebellar competition is also observed but is expressed in a converse manner. During high task demands over-activity is seen in the cerebellum, but non-responsiveness could be observed in prefrontal and limbic cortices. It seems that in addicts and heavy drug users the cerebellum controls functions normally managed by the prefrontal cortices. However, the cerebellum does not produce behavioral flexible executive control, but a rapid and automatic form of control. Perhaps, it is a part of the explanation why addicts show impairment in executive function and perseverative behavior. Tentatively, it is suggested that drug-induced cerebellar neuroplasticity, (e.g., sensitization of molecular parameters), may induce cerebellar hyper-responsiveness, where the vulnerability of the prefrontal cortex to be depressed by drugs of abuse is enhanced. Also, it is possible that drug-induced hypo-frontality smoothes the progress of cerebellar overactivation by drugs, or perhaps both processes could be produced in parallel.

Conclusion

The cerebellum is potentially a key modulator that impacts and is impacted by addiction. Specific structures in the posterior cerebellar hemispheres, such as hemispheric lobule VI and crus I, are particularly salient as contributing factors. One limitation in this feld of study is that addictive drugs affects multiple regions of the brain outside the cerebellum. Affected and connected areas may exert influences on cerebellar structures, making results difcult to interpret. Despite the existing dependency between different components of the nervous system, develepment of measuring instruments makes it possible to carry out more specific studies that specify the physiological relevance of the cerebellum to addiction.

As discussed in this review, chronic and excessive consumption of addictive drug leads to neuroanatomical alterations in the adult and/or fetal cerebellum, including neuronal loss and structural degradation. The exposure of these substances also triggers abnormal cerebellar activity. Since the cerebellum is decisively interposed to relate processing of exteroceptive and interoceptive stimuli to action [22, 23], drug induced "re-wiring" [24] of cerebellar circuitry may produce decisive functional consequences for behavior. In this regard, the common hypotheses suggest that drug induced activity-dependent synaptic changes in the cerebellum are central to transit from a pattern of recreational drug taking to a compulsive behavioral phenotype (Figure 6). Functional and structural modifications produced by drugs in the cerebellum may enhance the susceptibility of fronto-cerebellar circuitry to be changed by repeated drug exposure. As a part of this functional reorganization drug-induced cerebellar hyper-responsiveness appears to be central to reduce the influence of executive control of the prefrontal cortex on behavior and to transfer to an automatic mode of control. Thus, it can be expected the characteristic patterns of cerebellar hyperactivity and prefrontal hypoactivity to follow a temporal gradient, the cerebellum being more important as the exposure to drugs is repeated. In this sense, further animal studies is required to clarify if the cerebellum is implicated in the sensitization of the incentive salience effect and in the transition from a pattern of recreational drug taking to the compulsive behavioral phenotype. It is also crucial to depict how the cerebellar storage of long-term memory contributes to this transit and the subsequent relapse. Finally, it's required to know if the vulnerability of the prefrontal cortex to be impaired by drugs is related to cerebellar hyperactivity.

Specifically, if cerebellar vulnerability factors for addiction could be defined, they might be used to target susceptible individuals for early interventions. On the other hand, abnormalities arising in the context of ongoing addictive disorder may be used for diagnostic purposes and/or for a choice of a proper therapeutic agent in conjunction with monitoring of therapeutic response. The proposed hypothesis may also provide important leads for recognition and treatment of reward deficiency syndrome typical of patients with other disorders, where cerebellar abnormalities were also noted, including depression, schizophrenia and post-traumatic stress disorder.

References

[1] Weissbach, A; Werner, E; Bally, JF; Tunc, S; Löns, S; Timmann, D; Zeuner, KE; Tadic, V; Brüggemann, N; Lang, A; Klein, C. Alcohol

improves cerebellar learning deficit in myoclonus–dystonia: A clinical and electrophysiological investigation. *Annals of neurology,* 2017, Oct 1, 82(4), 543-53.

[2] Moulton, EA; Elman, I; Becerra, LR; Goldstein, RZ; Borsook, D. The cerebellum and addiction: insights gained from neuroimaging research. *Addiction biology,* 2014, May 1, 19(3), 317-31.

[3] Greer, TL; Thompson, LT. Eyeblink Classical Conditioning in Psychiatric Conditions: Novel Uses for a Classic Paradigm. *Frontiers in psychiatry,* 2017, Mar 27, 8, 48.

[4] Jörntell, H. Cerebellar physiology: links between microcircuitry properties and sensorimotor functions. *The Journal of physiology,* 2017, Jan 1, 595(1), 11-27.

[5] Voogd, J; Marani, E. Gross Anatomy of the Cerebellum. *In Essentials of Cerebellum and Cerebellar Disorders*, 2016 (pp. 33-38). Springer, Cham.

[6] Ito, M. Cerebellar microcomplexes. *In International review of neurobiology*, 1997 Jan 1, (Vol. *41*, pp. 475-487). Academic Press.

[7] Gao, Z; Van Beugen, BJ; De Zeeuw, CI. Distributed synergistic plasticity and cerebellar learning. *Nature Reviews Neuroscience*, 2012 Sep, 13(9), 619.

[8] Solouki, S; Pooyan, M. Arrangement and Applying of Movement Patterns in the Cerebellum Based on Semi-supervised Learning. *The Cerebellum*, 2016, Jun 1, 15(3), 299-305.

[9] Luque, NR; Garrido, JA; Naveros, F; Carrillo, RR; D'Angelo, E; Ros, E. Distributed cerebellar motor learning: a spike-timing-dependent plasticity model. *Frontiers in computational neuroscience,* 2016, Mar 2, 10, 17.

[10] D'Angelo, E; Nieus, T; Maffei, A; Armano, S; Rossi, P; Taglietti, V; Fontana, A; Naldi, G. Theta-frequency bursting and resonance in cerebellar granule cells: experimental evidence and modeling of a slow K+-dependent mechanism. *Journal of Neuroscience,* 2001 Feb 1, 21(3), 759-70.

[11] Chadderton, P; Margrie, TW; Häusser, M. Integration of quanta in cerebellar granule cells during sensory processing. *Nature*, 2004 Apr, 428(6985), 856.

[12] Bower, JM. The organization of cerebellar cortical circuitry revisited. *Annals of the New York Academy of Sciences,* 2002, Dec 1, 978(1), 135-55.

[13] Hirono, M; Yoshioka, T; Konishi, S. GABA B receptor activation enhances mGluR-mediated responses at cerebellar excitatory synapses. *Nature neuroscience,* 2001 Dec, 4(12), 1207.

[14] Batchelor, AM; Garthwaite, J. Novel synaptic potentials in cerebellar Purkenje cells: Probable mediation by metabotropic glutamate receptors. *Neuropharmacology*, 1993 Jan 1, 32(1), 11-20.

[15] Ito, M. Cerebellar circuitry as a neuronal machine. *Progress in neurobiology,* 2006, Apr 30, 78(3), 272-303.

[16] Simpson, JI; Wylie, DR; De Zeeuw, CI. On climbing fiber signals and their consequence (s). *Behavioral and Brain Sciences,* 1996 Sep, 19(3), 384-98.

[17] Ito, M. Mechanisms of motor learning in the cerebellum. *Brain research,* 2000, Dec 15, 886(1-2), 237-45.

[18] Bastian, AJ. Learning to predict the future: the cerebellum adapts feedforward movement control. *Current opinion in neurobiology*, 2006, Dec 1, 16(6), 645-9.

[19] Ito, M; Sakurai, M; Tongroach, P. Climbing fibre induced depression of both mossy fibre responsiveness and glutamate sensitivity of cerebellar Purkinje cells. *The Journal of Physiology*, 1982, Mar 1, 324(1), 113-34.

[20] Sakurai, M. Synaptic modification of parallel fibre-Purkinje cell transmission in *in vitro* guinea-pig cerebellar slices. *The Journal of Physiology*, 1987, Dec 1, 394(1), 463-80.

[21] Safo, PK; Regehr, WG. Endocannabinoids control the induction of cerebellar LTD. *Neuron*, 2005, Nov 23, 48(4), 647-59.

[22] Miquel, M; Toledo, R; García, LI; Coria-Avila, GA; Manzo, J. Why should we keep the cerebellum in mind when thinking about addiction?. *Current drug abuse reviews*, 2009, Jan 1, 2(1), 26-40.

[23] Anderson, CM; Maas, LC; deB Frederick, B; Bendor, JT; Spencer, TJ; Livni, E; Lukas, SE; Fischman, AJ; Madras, BK; Renshaw, PF; Kaufman, MJ. Cerebellar vermis involvement in cocaine-related behaviors. *Neuropsychopharmacology*, 2006 Jun, 31(6), 1318.

[24] Wolf, ME; Sun, X; Mangiavacchi, S; Chao, SZ. Psychomotor stimulants and neuronal plasticity. *Neuropharmacology*, 2004, Jan 1, 47, 61-79.

[25] Goodman, A. Addiction: definition and implications. *Addiction*, 1990, Nov 1, 85(11), 1403-8.

[26] West, R. Theories of addiction. *Addiction*, 2001 Jan, 96(1), 3-13.

[27] Hyman, SE; Malenka, RC; Nestler, EJ. Neural mechanisms of addiction: the role of reward-related learning and memory. *Annu. Rev. Neurosci*, 2006, Jul 21, 29, 565-98.

[28] Hyman, SE. Addiction: a disease of learning and memory. *American Journal of Psychiatry,* 2005, Aug 1, 162(8), 1414-22.

[29] Fillmore, MT. Acute alcohol-induced impairment of cognitive functions: past and present findings. *International Journal on Disability and Human Development,* 2007, 6(2), 115-26.

[30] Gilpin, NW; Koob, GF. Neurobiology of alcohol dependence: focus on motivational mechanisms. *Alcohol Research & Health*, 2008, 31(3), 185.

[31] Yokota, O; Tsuchiya, K; Terada, S; Oshima, K; Ishizu, H; Matsushita, M; Kuroda, S; Akiyama, H. Frequency and clinicopathological characteristics of alcoholic cerebellar degeneration in Japan: a cross-sectional study of 1,509 postmortems. *Acta neuropathologica*, 2006, Jul 1, 112(1), 43-51.

[32] Chanraud, S; Martelli, C; Delain, F; Kostogianni, N; Douaud, G; Aubin, HJ; Reynaud, M; Martinot, JL. Brain morphometry and cognitive performance in detoxified alcohol-dependents with preserved psychosocial functioning. *Neuropsychopharmacology*, 2007 Feb, 32(2), 429.

[33] Belmeguenai, A; Botta, P; Weber, JT; Carta, M; De Ruiter, M; De Zeeuw, CI; Valenzuela, CF; Hansel, C. Alcohol impairs long-term

depression at the cerebellar parallel fiber–Purkinje cell synapse. *Journal of neurophysiology,* 2008 Dec, 100(6), 3167-74.

[34] Luo, J. *Effects of ethanol on the cerebellum: advances and prospects*, 2015, 383-85.

[35] Lovinger, DM; White, G; Weight, FF. Ethanol inhibits NMDA-activated ion current in hippocampal neurons. *Science*, 1989, Mar 31, 243(4899), 1721-4.

[36] Piochon, C; Irinopoulou, T; Brusciano, D; Bailly, Y; Mariani, J; Levenes, C. NMDA receptor contribution to the climbing fiber response in the adult mouse Purkinje cell. *Journal of Neuroscience,* 2007, Oct 3, 27(40), 10797-809.

[37] Carta, M; Mameli, M; Valenzuela, CF. Alcohol potently modulates climbing fiber→ Purkinje neuron synapses: role of metabotropic glutamate receptors. *Journal of Neuroscience*, 2006, Feb 15, 26(7), 1906-12.

[38] Jörntell, H; Hansel, C. Synaptic memories upside down: bidirectional plasticity at cerebellar parallel fiber-Purkinje cell synapses. *Neuron*, 2006, Oct 19, 52(2), 227-38.

[39] Servais, L; Hourez, R; Bearzatto, B; Gall, D; Schiffmann, SN; Cheron, G. Purkinje cell dysfunction and alteration of long-term synaptic plasticity in fetal alcohol syndrome. *Proceedings of the National Academy of Sciences,* 2007, Jun 5, 104(23), 9858-63.

[40] Gruol, DL; Parsons, KL; DiJulio, N. Acute ethanol alters calcium signals elicited by glutamate receptor agonists and K+ depolarization in cultured cerebellar Purkinje neurons. *Brain research,* 1997, Oct 31, 773(1-2), 82-9.

[41] Sanna, PP; Simpson, C; Lutjens, R; Koob, G. ERK regulation in chronic ethanol exposure and withdrawal. *Brain research*, 2002, Sep 6, 948(1-2), 186-91.

[42] Barco, A; Bailey, CH; Kandel, ER. Common molecular mechanisms in explicit and implicit memory. *Journal of neurochemistry*, 2006, Jun 1, 97(6), 1520-33.

[43] Asher, O; Cunningham, TD; Yao, L; Gordon, AS; Diamond, I. Ethanol stimulates cAMP-responsive element (CRE)-mediated

transcription via CRE-binding protein and cAMP-dependent protein kinase. *Journal of pharmacology and experimental therapeutics,* 2002, Apr 1, 301(1), 66-70.

[44] Light, KE; Hayar, AM; Pierce, DR. Electrophysiological and immunohistochemical evidence for an increase in GABAergic inputs and HCN channels in Purkinje cells that survive developmental ethanol exposure. *The Cerebellum,* 2015, Aug 1, 14(4), 398-412.

[45] Lindquist, DH; Sokoloff, G; Milner, E; Steinmetz, JE. Neonatal ethanol exposure results in dose-dependent impairments in the acquisition and timing of the conditioned eye blink response and altered cerebellar interpositus nucleus and hippocampal CA1 unit activity in adult rats. *Alcohol,* 2013, Sep 1, 47(6), 447-57.

[46] Servais, L; Bearzatto, B; Delvaux, V; Noël, E; Leach, R; Brasseur, M; Schiffmann, SN; Guy, C. Effect of chronic ethanol ingestion on Purkinje and Golgi cell firing *in vivo* and on motor coordination in mice. *Brain research,* 2005, Sep 7, 1055(1-2), 171-9.

[47] Diwadkar, VA; Meintjes, EM; Goradia, D; Dodge, NC; Warton, C; Molteno, CD; Jacobson, SW; Jacobson, JL. Differences in cortico-striatal-cerebellar activation during working memory in syndromal and nonsyndromal children with prenatal alcohol exposure. *Human brain mapping,* 2013, Aug 1, 34(8), 1931-45.

[48] Parks, MH; Morgan, VL; Pickens, DR; Price, RR; Dietrich, MS; Nickel, MK; Martin, PR. Brain fMRI activation associated with self-paced finger tapping in chronic alcohol-dependent patients. *Alcoholism: Clinical and Experimental Research,* 2003, Apr 1, 27(4), 704-11.

[49] du Plessis, L; Jacobson, SW; Molteno, CD; Robertson, FC; Peterson, BS; Jacobson, JL; Meintjes, EM. Neural correlates of cerebellar-mediated timing during finger tapping in children with fetal alcohol spectrum disorders. *Neuro Image: Clinical,* 2015, Jan 1, 7, 562-70.

[50] Victor, M; ADAMS, RD; Mancall, EL. A restricted form of cerebellar cortical degeneration occurring in alcoholic patients. *AMA Archives of Neurology,* 1959, Dec 1, 1(6), 579-688.

[51] Dikranian, K; Qin, YQ; Labruyere, J; Nemmers, B; Olney, JW. Ethanol-induced neuroapoptosis in the developing rodent cerebellum and related brain stem structures. *Developmental Brain Research,* 2005, Mar 22, 155(1), 1-3.

[52] Paula-Barbosa, MM; Tavares, MA. Long term alcohol consumption induces microtubular changes in the adult rat cerebellar cortex. *Brain research,* 1985, Jul 22, 339(1), 195-9.

[53] Tavares, MA; Paula-Barbosa, MM; Gray, EG. A morphometric Golgi analysis of the Purkinje cell dendritic tree after long-term alcohol consumption in the adult rat. *Journal of neurocytology*, 1983, Dec 1, 12(6), 939-48.

[54] Tavares, MA; Paula-Barbosa, MM; Cadete-Leite, A. Morphological evidence of climbing fiber plasticity after long-term alcohol intake. *Neurobehavioral toxicology and teratology,* 1986, 8(5), 481-5.

[55] Sullivan, EV; Deshmukh, A; Desmond, JE; Mathalon, DH; Rosenbloom, MJ; Lim, KO; Pfefferbaum, A. Contribution of alcohol abuse to cerebellar volume deficits in men with schizophrenia. *Archives of general psychiatry,* 2000, Sep 1, 57(9), 894-902.

[56] Spottiswoode, BS; Meintjes, EM; Anderson, AW; Molteno, CD; Stanton, ME; Dodge, NC; Gore, JC; Peterson, BS; Jacobson, JL; Jacobson, SW. Diffusion tensor imaging of the cerebellum and eye blink conditioning in fetal alcohol spectrum disorder. *Alcoholism: Clinical and Experimental Research,* 2011, Dec 1, 35(12), 2174-83.

[57] Mattson, SN; Riley, EP; Jernigan, TL; Garcia, A; Kaneko, WM; Ehlers, CL; Jones, KL. A decrease in the size of the basal ganglia following prenatal alcohol exposure: a preliminary report. *Neuro-toxicology and teratology,* 1994, May 1, 16(3), 283-9.

[58] Chanraud, S; Reynaud, M; Wessa, M; Penttilä, J; Kostogianni, N; Cachia, A; Artiges, E; Delain, F; Perrin, M; Aubin, HJ; Cointepas, Y. Diffusion tensor tractography in mesencephalic bundles: relation to mental flexibility in detoxified alcohol-dependent subjects. *Neuro-psychopharmacology*, 2009 Apr, 34(5), 1223.

[59] Autti-Rämö, I; Autti, T; Korkman, M; Kettunen, S; Salonen, O; Valanne, L. MRI findings in children with school problems who had

been exposed prenatally to alcohol. *Developmental medicine and child neurology,* 2002 Feb, 44(2), 98-106.

[60] Cheng, DT; Jacobson, SW; Jacobson, JL; Molteno, CD; Stanton, ME; Desmond, JE. Eyeblink classical conditioning in alcoholism and fetal alcohol spectrum disorders. *Frontiers in psychiatry,* 2015, Nov 2, 6, 155.

[61] Oomah, BD; Busson, M; Godfrey, DV; Drover, JC. Characteristics of hemp (*Cannabis sativa* L.) seed oil. *Food chemistry*, 2002, Jan 1, 76(1), 33-43.

[62] Casu, MA; Pisu, C; Sanna, A; Tambaro, S; Spada, GP; Mongeau, R; Pani, L. Effect of Δ9-tetrahydrocannabinol on phosphorylated CREB in rat cerebellum: An immunohistochemical study. *Brain research,* 2005, Jun 28, 1048(1-2), 41-7.

[63] Viganò, D; Cascio, MG; Rubino, T; Fezza, F; Vaccani, A; Di Marzo, V; Parolaro, D. Chronic morphine modulates the contents of the endocannabinoid, 2-arachidonoyl glycerol, in rat brain. *Neuropsychopharmacology*, 2003 Jun, 28(6), 1160.

[64] Vinod, KY; Yalamanchili, R; Xie, S; Cooper, TB; Hungund, BL. Effect of chronic ethanol exposure and its withdrawal on the endocannabinoid system. *Neurochemistry international,* 2006, Nov 1, 49(6), 619-25.

[65] Basavarajappa, BS; Hungund, BL. Role of the endocannabinoid system in the development of tolerance to alcohol. *Alcohol and alcoholism,* 2004, Nov 18, 40(1), 15-24.

[66] Cousijn, J; Wiers, RW; Ridderinkhof, KR; van den Brink, W; Veltman, DJ; Goudriaan, AE. Grey matter alterations associated with cannabis use: results of a VBM study in heavy cannabis users and healthy controls. *Neuroimage*, 2012, Feb 15, 59(4), 3845-51.

[67] Sim, ME; Lyoo, IK; Streeter, CC; Covell, J; Sarid-Segal, O; Ciraulo, DA; Kim, MJ; Kaufman, MJ; Yurgelun-Todd, DA; Renshaw, PF. Cerebellar gray matter volume correlates with duration of cocaine use in cocaine-dependent subjects. *Neuropsychopharmacology*, 2007 Oct, 32(10), 2229.

[68] Barrós-Loscertales, A; Garavan, H; Bustamante, JC; Ventura-Campos, N; Llopis, JJ; Belloch, V; Parcet, MA; Ávila, C. Reduced striatal volume in cocaine-dependent patients. *Neuroimage*, 2011, Jun 1, 56(3), 1021-6.

[69] Schmahmann, JD; Sherman, JC. The cerebellar cognitive affective syndrome. *Brain: a journal of neurology,* 1998, Apr 1, 121(4), 561-79.

[70] Kalivas, PW; Volkow, ND. The neural basis of addiction: a pathology of motivation and choice. *American Journal of Psychiatry,* 2005, Aug 1, 162(8), 1403-13.

[71] Vazquez-Sanroman, D; Carbo-Gas, M; Leto, K; Cerezo-Garcia, M; Gil-Miravet, I; Sanchis-Segura, C; Carulli, D; Rossi, F; Miquel, M. Cocaine-induced plasticity in the cerebellum of sensitised mice. *Psychopharmacology*, 2015, Dec 1, 232(24), 4455-67.

[72] Schadrack, J; Willoch, F; Platzer, S; Bartenstein, P; Mahal, B; Dworzak, D; Wester, HJ; Zieglgänsberger, W; Tölle, TR. Opioid receptors in the human cerebellum: evidence from [11C] diprenorphine PET, mRNA expression and autoradiography. *Neuroreport*, 1999, Feb 25, 10(3), 619-24.

[73] Walhovd, KB; Moe, V; Slinning, K; Due-Tønnessen, P; Bjørnerud, A; Dale, AM; Van der Kouwe, A; Quinn, BT; Kosofsky, B; Greve, D; Fischl, B. Volumetric cerebral characteristics of children exposed to opiates and other substances in utero. *Neuroimage*, 2007, Jul 15, 36(4), 1331-44.

[74] Bora, E; Yücel, M; Fornito, A; Pantelis, C; Harrison, BJ; Cocchi, L; Pell, G; Lubman, DI. White matter microstructure in opiate addiction. *Addiction biology*, 2012, Jan 1, 17(1), 141-8.

[75] Saal, D; Dong, Y; Bonci, A; Malenka, RC. Drugs of abuse and stress trigger a common synaptic adaptation in dopamine neurons. *Neuron*, 2003, Feb 20, 37(4), 577-82.

[76] Brown, LF; Kroenke, K; Theobald, DE; Wu, J; Tu, W. The association of depression and anxiety with health-related quality of life in cancer patients with depression and/or pain. *Psycho-Oncology,* 2010, Jul 1, 19(7), 734-41.

[77] Nugent, FS; Penick, EC; Kauer, JA. Opioids block long-term potentiation of inhibitory synapses. *Nature*, 2007, Apr, 446(7139), 1086.

[78] Nugent, FS; Niehaus, JL; Kauer, JA. PKG and PKA signaling in LTP at GABAergic synapses. *Neuropsychopharmacology*, 2009 Jun, 34(7), 1829.

[79] Wang, GJ; Volkow, ND; Logan, J; Pappas, NR; Wong, CT; Zhu, W; Netusll, N; Fowler, JS. Brain dopamine and obesity. *The Lancet*, 2001, Feb 3, 357(9253), 354-7.

[80] Melchitzky, DS; Lewis, DA. Tyrosine hydroxylase-and dopamine transporter-immunoreactive axons in the primate cerebellum. *Neuropsychopharmacology*, 2000 May, 22(5), 466.

[81] Klitenick, MA; Tham, CS; Fibiger, HC. Cocaine and d-amphetamine increase c-fos expression in the rat cerebellum. *Synapse*, 1995, Jan 1, 19(1), 29-36.

[82] Carlezon, Jr. WA; Nestler, E. Elevated levels of GluR1 in the midbrain: a trigger for sensitization to drugs of abuse? *Trends in neurosciences*, 2002, Dec 1, 25(12), 610-5.

[83] Berridge, KC; Robinson, TE. Liking, wanting, and the incentive-sensitization theory of addiction. *American Psychologist,* 2016 Nov, 71(8), 670.

[84] Robinson, TE; Berridge, KC. The psychology and neurobiology of addiction: an incentive–sensitization view. *Addiction*, 2000, Aug 1, 95(8s2), 91-117.

[85] Everitt, BJ; Robbins, TW. Neural systems of reinforcement for drug addiction: from actions to habits to compulsion. *Nature neuroscience,* 2005 Nov, 8(11), 1481.

[86] Vezina, P. Sensitization of midbrain dopamine neuron reactivity and the self-administration of psychomotor stimulant drugs. *Neuroscience & Biobehavioral Reviews,* 2004, Jan 1, 27(8), 827-39.

[87] De Fonseca, FR; Gorriti, MA; Fernandez-Ruiz, JJ; Palomo, T; Ramos, JA. Downregulation of rat brain cannabinoid binding sites after chronic Δ9-tetrahydrocannabinol treatment. *Pharmacology Biochemistry and Behavior,* 1994, Jan 1, 47(1), 33-40.

[88] Miquel, M; Font, L; Sanchis-Segura, C; Aragon, CM. Neonatal administration of monosodium glutamate prevents the development of ethanol-but not psychostimulant-induced sensitization: a putative role of the arcuate nucleus. *European Journal of Neuroscience*, 2003, May 1, 17(10), 2163-70.

[89] Bhargava, HN; Kumar, S. Sensitization to the locomotor stimulant effect of cocaine modifies the binding of [3H] MK-801 to brain regions and spinal cord of the mouse. *General Pharmacology: The Vascular System*, 1999, Mar 1, 32(3), 359-63.

[90] Couceyro, P; Pollock, KM; Drews, K; Douglass, J. Cocaine differentially regulates activator protein-1 mRNA levels and DNA-binding complexes in the rat striatum and cerebellum. *Molecular pharmacology,* 1994, Oct 1, 46(4), 667-76.

[91] Barik, S; de Beaurepaire, R. Dopamine D3 modulation of locomotor activity and sleep in the nucleus accumbens and in lobules 9 and 10 of the cerebellum in the rat. *Progress in Neuro-Psychopharmacology and Biological Psychiatry*, 2005, Jun 1, 29(5), 718-26.

[92] Lou, M; Wang, E; Shen, Y; Wang, J. Cue-elicited craving in heroin addicts at different abstinent time: an fMRI pilot study. *Substance use & misuse,* 2012, Apr 17, 47(6), 631-9.

[93] Schneider, F; Habel, U; Wagner, M; Franke, P; Salloum, JB; Shah, NJ; Toni, I; Sulzbach, C; Hönig, K; Maier, W; Gaebel, W. Subcortical correlates of craving in recently abstinent alcoholic patients. *American Journal of Psychiatry,* 2001, Jul 1, 158(7), 1075-83.

[94] Sell, LA; Morris, JS; Bearn, J; Frackowiak, RS; Friston, KJ; Dolan, RJ. Neural responses associated with cue evoked emotional states and heroin in opiate addicts. *Drug & Alcohol Dependence*, 2000, Aug 1, 60(2), 207-16.

[95] Kilts, CD; Schweitzer, JB; Quinn, CK; Gross, RE; Faber, TL; Muhammad, F; Ely, TD; Hoffman, JM; Drexler, KP. Neural activity related to drug craving in cocaine addiction. *Archives of general psychiatry*, 2001, Apr 1, 58(4), 334-41.

[96] Volkow, ND; Wang, GJ; Ma, Y; Fowler, JS; Zhu, W; Maynard, L; Telang, F; Vaska, P; Ding, YS; Wong, C; Swanson, JM. Expectation

enhances the regional brain metabolic and the reinforcing effects of stimulants in cocaine abusers. *Journal of neuroscience,* 2003, Dec 10, 23(36), 11461-8.

[97] Dum, RP; Strick, PL. An unfolded map of the cerebellar dentate nucleus and its projections to the cerebral cortex. *Journal of neurophysiology,* 2003, Jan 1, 89(1), 634-9.

[98] Berlin, HA; Rolls, ET; Kischka, U. Impulsivity, time perception, emotion and reinforcement sensitivity in patients with orbitofrontal cortex lesions. *Brain*, 2004, May 1, 127(5), 1108-26.

[99] Anand, BK; Malhotra, CL; Singh, B; Dua, S. Cerebellar projections to limbic system. *Journal of neurophysiology,* 1959, Jul 1, 22(4), 451-7.

[100] Snider, RS; Maiti, A. Cerebellar contributions to the Papez circuit. *Journal of neuroscience research,* 1976, Jan 1, 2(2), 133-46.

[101] Marcinkiewicz, M; Morcos, R; Chretien, MC. CNS connections with the median raphe nucleus: Retrograde tracing with WGA-apoHRP-gold complex in the rat. *Journal of Comparative Neurology*, 1989, Nov 1, 289(1), 11-35.

[102] Paradiso, S; Robinson, RG; Boles Ponto, LL; Watkins, GL; Hichwa, RD. Regional cerebral blood flow changes during visually induced subjective sadness in healthy elderly persons. *The Journal of neuropsychiatry and clinical neurosciences,* 2003 Feb, 15(1), 35-44.

[103] Goel, V; Dolan, RJ. The functional anatomy of humor: segregating cognitive and affective components. *Nature neuroscience,* 2001 Mar, 4(3), 237.

[104] Schmahmann, JD; Caplan, D. Cognition, emotion and the cerebellum. *Brain*, 2006 Feb 1, 129(2), 290-2.

[105] Grant, S; London, ED; Newlin, DB; Villemagne, VL; Liu, X; Contoreggi, C; Phillips, RL; Kimes, AS; Margolin, A. Activation of memory circuits during cue-elicited cocaine craving. *Proceedings of the National Academy of Sciences,* 1996 Oct 15, 93(21), 12040-5.

[106] Bonson, KR; Grant, SJ; Contoreggi, CS; Links, JM; Metcalfe, J; Weyl, HL; Kurian, V; Ernst, M; London, ED. Neural systems and cue-

induced cocaine craving. *Neuropsychopharmacology*, 2002 Mar, 26(3), 376.

[107] Duvauchelle, CL; Ikegami, A; Asami, S; Robens, J; Kressin, K; Castaneda, E. Effects of cocaine context on NAcc dopamine and behavioral activity after repeated intravenous cocaine administration. *Brain research,* 2000 Apr 17, 862(1-2), 49-58.

[108] Hemby, SE; Koves, TR; Smith, JE; Dworkin, SI. Differences in extracellular dopamine concentrations in the nucleus accumbens during response-dependent and response-independent cocaine administration in the rat. *Psychopharmacology*, 1997, Sep 1, 133(1), 7-16.

[109] Hubert, V; Beaunieux, H; Chételat, G; Platel, H; Landeau, B; Danion, JM; Viader, F; Desgranges, B; Eustache, F. The dynamic network subserving the three phases of cognitive procedural learning. *Human brain mapping,* 2007 Dec, 28(12), 1415-29.

[110] Fliessbach, K; Trautner, P; Quesada, CM; Elger, CE; Weber, B. Cerebellar contributions to episodic memory encoding as revealed by fMRI. *Neuroimage*, 2007, Apr 15, 35(3), 1330-7.

[111] Snider, RS; Maiti, A; Snider, SR. Cerebellar pathways to ventral midbrain and nigra. *Experimental neurology*, 1976, Dec 1, 53(3), 714-28.

[112] Schweighofer, N; Doya, K; Kuroda, S. Cerebellar aminergic neuromodulation: towards a functional understanding. *Brain Research Reviews*, 2004, Mar 1, 44(2-3), 103-16.

[113] Buck, R. The biological affects: a typology. *Psychological review*, 1999 Apr, 106(2), 301.

[114] Papez, JW. A proposed mechanism of emotion. *Archives of Neurology & Psychiatry,* 1937, Oct 1, 38(4), 725-43.

[115] Frijda, NH. *The emotions.* Cambridge University Press, 1986.

[116] Jentsch, JD; Taylor, JR. Impulsivity resulting from frontostriatal dysfunction in drug abuse: implications for the control of behavior by reward-related stimuli. *Psychopharmacology*, 1999, Oct 1, 146(4), 373-90.

[117] Bechara, A. Decision making, impulse control and loss of willpower to resist drugs: a neurocognitive perspective. *Nature neuroscience*, 2005 Nov, 8(11), 1458.

[118] Volkow, ND; Fowler, JS; Wang, GJ. The addicted human brain viewed in the light of imaging studies: brain circuits and treatment strategies. *Neuropharmacology*, 2004, Jan 1, 47, 3-13.

[119] Montague, PR; Hyman, SE; Cohen, JD. Computational roles for dopamine in behavioural control. *Nature*, 2004, Oct 13, 431(7010), 760.

[120] Goldstein, RZ; Volkow, ND. Dysfunction of the prefrontal cortex in addiction: neuroimaging findings and clinical implications. *Nature reviews neuroscience,* 2011 Nov, 12(11), 652.

[121] Strick, PL; Dum, RP; Fiez, JA. Cerebellum and nonmotor function. *Annual review of neuroscience*, 2009, Jul 21, 32, 413-34.

[122] Kelly, RM; Strick, PL. Cerebellar loops with motor cortex and prefrontal cortex of a nonhuman primate. *Journal of neuroscience*, 2003, Sep 10, 23(23), 8432-44.

[123] Ito, M. Control of mental activities by internal models in the cerebellum. *Nature Reviews Neuroscience,* 2008 Apr, 9(4), 304.

[124] Hester, R; Garavan, H. Executive dysfunction in cocaine addiction: evidence for discordant frontal, cingulate, and cerebellar activity. *Journal of Neuroscience*, 2004 Dec 8, 24(49), 11017-22.

[125] Desmond, JE; Chen, SA; DeRosa, E; Pryor, MR; Pfefferbaum, A; Sullivan, EV. Increased frontocerebellar activation in alcoholics during verbal working memory: an fMRI study. *Neuroimage*, 2003 Aug 1, 19(4), 1510-20.

[126] Bolla, KI; Eldreth, DA; Matochik, JA; Cadet, JL. Neural substrates of faulty decision-making in abstinent marijuana users. *Neuroimage*, 2005 Jun 1, 26(2), 480-92.

[127] Martin-Sölch, C; Magyar, S; Künig, G; Missimer, J; Schultz, W; Leenders, K. Changes in brain activation associated with reward processing in smokers and nonsmokers. *Experimental Brain Research*, 2001, Aug 1, 139(3), 278-86.

In: Development of the Cerebellum
Editor: Severina Fabbri
ISBN: 978-1-53614-317-1

Chapter 4

GECKO CEREBELLUM AFTER A LONG-TERM SPACEFLIGHT DURING THE "BION-M1" SPACE MISSION

A. S. Kharlamova, A. E. Proshchina, V. I. Gulimova, V. M. Barabanov, O. A. Junemann and S. V. Saveliev
Research Institute of Human Morphology, Moscow, Russia

ABSTRACT

In humans and other vertebrates, alterations in vestibular and motor function, including changes in linear vestibular-ocular reflexes, postural control systems, and so on, have been described under spaceflight conditions. Cerebellar structures are proposed to be involved in vestibular and locomotor disturbances in weightlessness.

The gecko (*Chondrodactylus turneri* GRAY 1864) is a prospective animal model for a spaceflight experiment. Geckos demonstrate effective adaptation to weightlessness, quickly attaching themselves to surfaces by means of their subdigital pads, and during the spaceflight they retain both attached positions and normal locomotion, showing normal foraging, exploratory, social, and even play behavior.

The cerebella of the thick-toed geckos after a 30-day spaceflight aboard "Bion-M1" biosatellite were examined and compared with terrarium and delayed synchronous control groups. Immunohistochemical and classical histological methods were used to reveal cell types in the anterior and posterior (vestibular) cerebellum.

In general, the histological appearance of the cerebellum was normal in all groups of geckos. However, some pathomorphological changes in the Purkinje cells (such as chromatolysis, vacuolization, and hyper-chromatosis) were detected. These cytomorphological features are a manifestation of the *in vivo* state of neurons, which correlates with the level of metabolism. A significant increase in the number of Purkinje cells with such changes were revealed only in the posterior vestibular cerebella of the geckos from the flight group in comparison with the control groups. It is reasonable to speculate that these changes detected in vestibular cerebellum Purkinje cells of geckos were caused by functional loading on the cells of this type during the spaceflight.

Similar data were obtained during the Purkinje cell study using neuron-specific beta-III-tubulin (NST) immunohistochemistry. Immuno-reactivity to NST was heterogeneous (decreasing in some cases and increasing in others) in Purkinje cells of the vestibular cerebellum of animals from all groups. An increase in the number of Purkinje cells with an altered NST immunoreactivity was revealed in the flight group. We did not identify any significant differences in the distribution and NST immunoreactivity of Purkinje cells in anterior cerebellum between flight and control groups of geckos.

The density of Purkinje cell dendrites was also measured in the molecular layer of the anterior and posterior cerebellum. There were no statistically significant alterations of the dendrite density between groups both in the anterior and posterior cerebellum.

The data coincide with the gecko behavior during the spaceflight, which was described in the "Bion-M1" space mission project. We propose that the nervous system is able to compensate for incorrect information from the vestibular system, using tactile and visual signals.

The gecko is a prospective animal model to enable study of the cerebellum of vertebrates after a spaceflight due to the relative simplicity of its organization and, at the same time, its similarities with other vertebrates.

Keywords: cerebellum, Purkinje cell, reptiles, spaceflight, weightlessness

1. INTRODUCTION

1.1. Cerebellum of Reptiles

Reptiles represent a basic cerebellar structure for terrestrial vertebrates. The base structure of the cerebellum, including primary (from vestibular ganglion), secondary (via vestibular nuclei) and tertiary (via the inferior olive) vestibular projections, is conservative within all vertebrates. The principal cytoarchitecture of the main neuronal and glial types of the cerebellar cortex is also similar in different vertebrate taxa (Barmack, 2003; Voogd and Glickstein, 1998). Thus, the reptile cerebellum seems to be a useful model object due to it is simplicity, on one hand, and because it presents the same key structure as mammals, on the other.

The vertebrate cerebellum is a dorsal outgrowth of the first rhombomere arising as paired enlages of the alar plate of the anterior rhombencephalon. The reptilian cerebellum consists of corpus cerebelli and small flocculus (also known as *auriculi* or auricular lobes). Cerebellar nuclei (medial and lateral) are described for lizards as a cell mass with an indistinct border located in the base of the lateral part of the corpus cerebelli. The corpus cerebelli can be divided into median (*pars interposita*) and lateral (*pars lateralis*) zones (Larsell, 1926). According to Larsell, the median zone is concerned with axial musculature movements and the lateral with limbs. The median zone seems to be homologous with the vermal zone of the mammalian cerebellum, and the lateral with the paravermal one (Goodman, 1964). In terms of the fibre connections, the posterior part of the corpus cerebelli seems to correspond with a nodular zone of mammals. Small reptilian auriculi are a mammalian floccular lobe homologue and have vestibular connections (Larsell, 1926). Reptilian flocculi arise between the lateral part of the cerebellar base and the primary vestibular region of rhombencephalon and are separated from the corpus cerebelli by a posterolateral fissure which also occurs in mammalian cerebellum. There are two primary sulci –anterior and posterior– which divide the cerebellum into anterior-, medius-, and posterior-lobes in the most developed among reptiles, the crocodilian cerebellum. It is considered that the sulcus anterior is the *fissura prima* homologue and the posterior is the *fissura secunda* of mammals (Larsell, 1947).

The reptilian cerebellar cortex, as in other vertebrates including mammals, comprises three layers: molecular, Purkinje cells, and granular. In many lizards, including the thick-toed gecko, the cerebellum is everted. The Purkinje cells are the main output neurons. Three longitudinal zones of Purkinje cells in each half of the cerebellum are distinguished: medial, intermediate, and lateral. These can be separated from each other by sparse of cell-free ranges. As in other vertebrates, reptiles have mossy and climbing afferent fibres. Along with the granular and Purkinje cells, they arrange the main cerebellar circuits.

The largest part of the afferent cerebellar inputs arise from rhombencephalon, including massive afferents from primary vestibular nuclei (and vestibular ganglion) and inferior olive (secondary vestibular structure) (Figure 1). Both primary and secondary vestibular projections have been demonstrated in reptiles (Bangma and ten Donkelaar, 1982). In reptiles, vestibular inputs mainly project into the lateral and intermediate (including inputs from vestibular ganglion) and auricular zones (Bangma and ten Donkelaar, 1982). The cerebellar efferents mostly project to the cerebellar nuclei, the red nucleus of the mesencephalon, vestibular nuclei, and the reticular formation of the rhombencephalon. Corticovestibular projections are mainly derived from the Purkinje cells from lateral medial and intermediate (vermal) and lateral (paravermal) zonesof the posterior lobe of the cerebellum (Goodman and Simpson, 1960), and from floccular, lateral, and intermediate zones, according to Bangma and ten Donkelaar's HRPstudy (1983, 1984).

Several forms of astrocytes exist in the cerebellar cortex of vertebrates. Radial glia participate in neuroblast migration during embryogenesis and are almost absent in adult mammals, while in lower terrestrial vertebrates, including reptiles, radial glial cells present postnatally (Lazzari and Franceschini, 2001). Bergmann glial cells are a special population of radial glial cells of the cerebellum, which are retained in adult mammals. Bergmann glia is developmentally related to the radial glia, which guide the Purkinje cells and the granule cells from their origin to a definite position in the cerebellar cortex. Bergmann glial cell somata are located around Purkinje cells and their processes go through the molecular cerebellar layer to reach the meningeal surface of the cerebellum (Yamada and Watanabe, 2002). It is widely accepted that the main role of Bergmann glial cells is to support the multiple Purkinje cell dendrites, which are also found in the molecular layer. Furthermore, Bergmann glia inhibits the Purkinje cells and participates in GABA synaptic transmission and the formation and maturation (stabilization) of synapses (Riquelme et al., 2002).

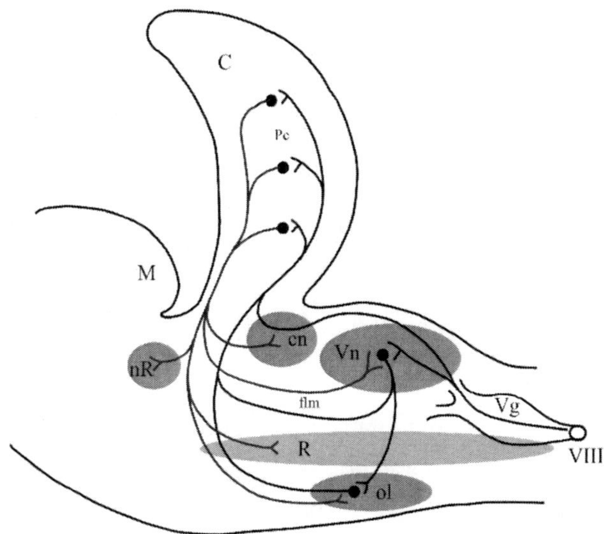

Figure 1. Scheme of the vestibular-cerebellar afferents and the main efferents of the reptilian cerebellum (for the full list of cerebellar connections see Larsell (1926), Nieuwenhuys (1967)). VIII – eight nerve (nervus statoacusticus), C – corpus cerebelli, cn – medial and lateral cerebellar nuclei, flm – fasciculus longitudinalis medialis, M – mesencephalon, ol – olive complex, Pc – Purkinje cell layer, R – reticular formation of the brainstem, nR – nucleus ruber, Vg – vestibular ganglion, Vn – vestibular nuclei complex.

1.2. Cerebellum in Space Research

Long-term spaceflight provides unique environmental conditions to which the vestibular system must adapt for optimal survival (Bruce, 2003).

In the conditions of spaceflight, the vestibular afferentation and the load on the locomotor apparatus are changed and the central nervous system needs to adapt to new conditions. (Anken and Rahmann, 1998; Minor, 1998). During spaceflight, the changed vestibular inputs from the inner ear need to be coordinated with the locomotor system signals and other sensory systems' afferentation. There are many studies regarding sensory conflicts in space (von Beckh, 1954; Mori, 1995; Wassersug et al., 2005; Kalb and Solomon, 2007). The vestibular system of vertebrates participates in short-term disturbances during microgravity and initial adaptation for weightlessness (Lichtenberg, 1988).

In humans and other vertebrates, space flight conditions cause alterations in vestibular and motor functions, including changes in linear vestibular-ocular reflexes and postural control systems, which induce fast motor reactions, such as posture perception and visual perception illusions, illusions of head movements and rotation, nystagmus, and vertigo and space motion sickness symptoms.

Astronauts demonstrate space adaptation syndrome, problems with spatial orientation, visual illusions, postural control disturbance, weakness and ataxia after landing (Thornton and Bonato, 2013; Kalb and Solomon, 2007; Slenzka, 2003). Sensorimotor adaptation to the changed vestibular afferentation and locomotor conditions in weightlessness gradually progress during spaceflight (Bruce, 2003; Koppelmans et al., 2016; Minor, 1998; Cohen et al., 2005). Readaptation after landing can take from several days to weeks (Koppelmans et al., 2016).

The functional and behavioral aspects of these short-term reversible changes are well studied. The physiological mechanisms underlying these effects are not clear. These changes are mostly related to the linear acceleration perception system without gravity and depend on the otolith apparatus. It has been hypothesized that a sensory conflict exists with the main role of the vestibular system (Oman and Cullen, 2014). For instance, space motion sickness symptoms are determined by linear acceleration perception. The adaptation to space flight induces motion illusion from head tilt (Young et al., 1984). In the central nervous system (CNS), inputs from the vestibular system are compared with visual and proprioceptive signals to control motions and compensate head and eye movements. Moreover, vestibulo-ocular reflex alterations during space flight correspond to disturbances in patients with cerebellar lesions (for details, see Bruce, 2003). Thus, alterations in the linear acceleration perception system, including the peripheral vestibular organ and CNS centres (primary and secondary vestibular centres of the brainstem and vestibular cerebellum) are primarily expected after long-term space flight.

It was shown that there are no severe non-reversible changes in the otolith organs of mammals due to weightlessness. Nevertheless, functional loading on the vestibular systems seems to increase during microgravity, which is evidenced from rat experiments. Morphological reversible changes were found in the peripheral part of the vestibular system (Ross, 1994, 2000) and changes in the vestibular cerebellum (Holstein et al., 1999) were observed. The amount of the synapses in the receptive part of the semicircular canals (Ross, 1994) and primary and secondary types of hair cells in the utricle macula were shown to increase during weightlessness and then decrease during readaptation after landing(Ross, 2000).

Vestibular centres have been poorly examined when compared with peripheral vestibular organs and behavioral changes (Cohen et al., 2005). Nevertheless, cerebellar structures seem to be also involved in vestibular and locomotor disturbance in weightlessness (Cohen et al., 2005; Krasnov and Krasnikov, 2009; Jamon, 2014). An increase of synapses was registered in the rhombencephalon *nucleus magnocellularis octavolateralis* in the fish *Xiphophorus helleri* (Ibsch et al., 2000). In the COSMOS biosatellite project, activity of the medial vestibular nucleus of primates was shown to increase in the first 5–7 days of spaceflight and then decrease (Cohen et al., 2005).

Cerebellar structures are also of interest due to their vestibular connections. Purkinje cell layer changes are the most frequently reported in spaceflight and altered gravity studies (Cohen et al., 2005; Holstein et al., 1999; Krasnov, 2008; Krasnov and Krasnikov, 2009). However, Purkinje cell influence over the vestibular and motion functions remains controversial. For instance, neurodegenerative changes of the Purkinje cells are described in rodents (Krasnov and Krasnikov, 2009); after 14days of spaceflight, cytochrome oxidase levels decreased in the molecular and Purkinje cell layers of the nodulus. These results were interpreted as evidence for the vestibular afferentation decreasing during spaceflight and, thus, functional activity reduction of the cells (Krasnov, 2008). These findings generally coincide with the results of the cerebellum experimental studies during altered gravity conditions (Sajdel-Sulkowska et al., 2005; Bruce, 2003). Other cerebellar structures, including the cerebellar glial cells, have been poorly studied during altered gravity and after space flights.

1.3. The Gecko as a Model Object for Space Research

The main problem of spaceflight studies of vertebrate model animals is the separation of weightlessness effects from associated stress. This is almost impossible and thus complicates analysis of the results. We supposed that the problem could be alleviated by using a model animal that is able to avoid flotation and thus become less stressed.

Some geckos possess a unique ability to attach and move on a variety of surfaces. The behavior of amphibians and reptiles, including six gecko species, was also studied during parabolic flights with short-term (up to 24 s) weightlessness (Wassersug et al., 2005). Reptile behavior varied from calm, slow movements in the case of amphisbaenians to violent and massive movements in the case of snakes, and body undulation and tail beating in terrestrial lizards. Arboreal geckos, as well as terrestrial ones, extend their limbs laterally, slightly inflecting the body dorsally and lifting their tails (i.e., assuming the skydiving posture), which increases their frontal surface area as if to increase drag and slow their free-fall speed in one-G. In addition, Wassersug and co-authors observed the gecko *Uroplatus* during weightlessness to be in contact with container surfaces; however, whether it was actively adhering to or passively in contact with the surfaces was not reported. Similar studies of long-term space experiments have not been realized to date.

We supposed that the adhesive gecko toes would allow them to attach to surfaces under conditions of weightlessness. The thick-toed geckos

(*Chondrodactylus turneri* GRAY 1864) were first proposed as a model object for space research in 2005. The geckos were successfully used in the research projects on board “Foton-M2” (2005), “Foton-M3” (2007), and “Bion-M1” (2013) satellites. In all aforementioned flights, there were no experimental animal deaths. Furthermore, thick-toed geckos seemed to demonstrate mainly normal behavior without severe symptoms associated with spaceflight, as discussed above (Khvatov et al., 2014; Barabanov et al., 2015; Proshchina et al., 2017). The gecko’s ability to be attached allowed the animals to maintain normal activity and behavior during most of the flight time. In the 12-day Foton-M3 orbital experiment, video recordings confirmed that thick-toed geckos preserved their ability to attach to surfaces and move more or less normally during a prolonged space experiment (Nikitin et al., 2008). In weightlessness, thick-toed geckos quickly restored attachment that was interrupted during take-off. They were also able to preserve normal activity, including locomotor, investigative, and social behavior. Another interesting finding of that flight was that a motionless (possibly sleeping) gecko was in free flotation for 13 min (Barabanov et al., 2018).

Histological examinations of the brains of geckos from the flight group revealed reversible structural cytological changes in the neurons of the rhombencephalon vestibular nuclei and motoneurons of the brain reticular formation, which were interpreted as signs of their metabolic activity enhancement (Proshchina et al., 2008). These data allowed us to hypothesize that the adhesion of gecko toes in weightlessness could be controlled by the nervous system, which could inhibit the inadequate vestibular inputs; however, in some cases this control becomes weaker or fails, leading to flotations.

Nevertheless, there were some doubts as to whether the revealed features in the geckos’ brain morphology and peculiarities of behavior during flotations were caused by factors related to spaceflight (Nikitin et al., 2008) or by poor housing conditions and life-support of the 12-day experiment on board Foton-M3 (small container, absence of food and water) (Almeida et al., 2006). Behavioral analysis of the results of the last 30-day experiment on board biosatellite “Bion-M1” confirms that the ability to attach to surfaces is an important factor in the gecko's adaptation to weightlessness. For most of the flight time (99.9%), the thick-toed geckos controlled their attachment to the surfaces and were able to preserve normal activity, including locomotor, feeding, investigative, social, and even play behavior (Barabanov et al., 2015). In weightlessness, they used all main forms of behavior evolved in Earth conditions, although they lost one mode of locomotion – the fast run. At the same time, having learned from their own experience during the first days of flight, the geckos acquired high accuracy in jumps in G0. Having adapted to new conditions, the geckos also demonstrated new behavioral reactions which are unusual for the Earth conditions, such as the detachment of some limbs from the surface while hanging in the air, rowing in the air to approach a chosen place of attachment, or ventral extension of limbs to find the substrate for attachment as a reflex reaction of the gecko awoken while floating. Flotations constituted a very small part of video registered flight time (0.1%). The geckos that were active and clearly awake became unattached when attempting to move or during locomotion, conflicts between geckos (fight or escape behavior, caused by the aggressive approach of another gecko), and intense engagement of geckos in communication activities (visual, tactile, or, probably, olfactory contacts). When geckos focused on external events or their own state, such as ingestion of a mealworm or shedding, this sometimes also led to the detachment of some or all of the limbs with subsequent flotation. Flotations of another registered type occurred in motionless (quiescent, (possibly sleeping) condition. The frequency of flotations in active (awake) geckos was highest in the first seven days of flight and dropped abruptly to isolated cases by the third and fourth weeks of flight, which suggests active neural control upon the geckos' attachment to the substrate and its enhancement during the adaptation of the CNS to weightlessness. The number of flotations for quiescent geckos (with reduced level of neural activity) was 4.5 times higher than that of the same animals in an active state and the frequency of such quiescent flotation remained high during the whole period of flight. The geckos which floated actively performed different actions to quickly restore attachment to the surface, such as assuming a skydiving posture or righting reflex, which were partially effective (Barabanov et al., 2018).

Mice are the classical subjects of space experiments. Mice have become the most prevalent 'mammalian model' in biomedical research (Cancedda et al., 2012; Andreev-Andrievskiy et al., 2014; Solomides et al., 2016). However, geckos also possess numerous advantages for the study of space biology and the study of geckos in the orbital experiment provides great interest and different perspectives. Due to its adhesion ability, gecko behavior in weightlessness differs a little from ground control and is similar to the behavior of mice in containers that are supplied with grating for attachment (Cancedda et al., 2012; Solomides et al., 2016). We speculate that this may reduce the stress on flotation, which allows us to distinguish the microgravity effect from the influences of hard continuous stress and to evaluate the real results of weightlessness. Additionally, geckos are less dependent on food and water compared with mammals and amphibians, which were used in similar previous experiments. It also transpires that geckos do not suffer from bone demineralization, characteristic of humans and other mammals after prolonged space flights (Saveliev et al., 2016). Before the start of our program, reptiles were rarely studied in continuous orbital experiments (Nikitin et al., 2008).

It is hypothesized that vestibular cerebellum could be involved in behavioral and functional changes and nervous system adaptations during spaceflight.

Reptiles demonstrate the basic structure of cerebellum for amniotes. The evolutionary old vestibular cerebellum is a stable structure among all terrestrial mammals, including the main vestibular afferent and efferent fibre connections. Reptiles also possess the same main neuronal and glial cerebellar cell types as mammals. In addition, the reptile cerebellum is simple in comparison with the foliated structure of higher vertebrates and, thus, is appropriate for model-based research.

Below, we provide results of the study of thick-toed gecko cerebellum after a 30-day experiment on board "Bion-M1".

2. Experiment Design

2.1. Animals and Life-Support

The experiment was conducted using adult virgin female thick-toed geckos (*Chondrodactylus turneri* GRAY 1864) aged 1.5–2 years under the guidelines for the use of live reptiles in research (approved by the Biomedicine Ethics Committee of the Russian Federation State Research Center Institute of Biomedical Problems, RAS (IBMP)/Physiology Section of the Russian Bioethics Committee of Russian Federation National Commission for UNESCO, Minute No. 319 from 4 April, 2013). The gecko females were chosen because male of thick-toed geckos can be aggressive towards each other, making it impossible to place more than one male in the same container; for statistical reasons it was necessary to have more than one gecko in a container. The average weight of the animals was 19.8 ± 1.7 g, the average snout-vent length was 79.2 ± 3.3mm, the average total length was 148.4 ± 9.1 mm, and the average brain weight was 95 mg.

Forty-five animals were used: 15 animals in the flight experiment (F), 15 animals as a delayed synchronous control (DSC) group, and 15 animals as a corresponding terrarium control (TC) group. The animals of the TC were housed under laboratory conditions (average day temperature 28^{0}C, average night temperature 24^{0}C). The geckos of the F and DSC groups were placed in containers, referred to here as the research and support blocks (RSB) with five females in each RSB. The F group was placed aboard the unmanned spacecraft, “Bion-M1”, for 30 days (near-circular orbit with an average height of 575 km and inclination 64.9°), which was launched on 19 April, 2013, and landed on 19 May, 2013. The RSB volume was 5.9 L. The walls were lined with hardboard (a type of fiber board) and the floor was textile laminate (a fabric-reinforced laminate). The RSB were equipped with five tubular shelters for geckos, a slot for a revolving-type feeder filled with food and drinking gel particles, two heating zones which created a local temperature of 31–32^{0}C on the floor surface during daytime, LEDs, a video camera, and a fan on the RSB cover (for details, see Barabanov et al., 2015). The DSC experiment was conducted after landing – from 25 July, 2013, to

26 August, 2013 – in the refurbished RSB. Geckos in the DSC were kept in the laboratory under conditions analogous to those experienced by the flight group. The RSB of the DSC were installed in a climatic chamber that replicated the temperature, humidity, and gas composition corresponding to flight-specific climate parameters.

2.2. Histology and Immunohistochemistry

Euthanasia of geckos was conducted by intraperitoneal injection of Nembutal. The dissection of FG geckos was performed within 13–16.5 h of the satellite landing. Gecko brains (whole) were acquired and fixed in 4% neutral buffered formalin (ph = 7,2-7,4). The samples were embedded in paraffin and then serial frontal and sagittal sections (10 mkm) were prepared. A series of each tenth section was prepared for the routine histology (cresyl violet (Nissl) and hematoxylin-eosin staining) and immune-histochemistry. All samples were processed simultaneously (from fixation to immunohistochemistry), to provide the same conditions for every sample.

We used a standard streptavidin–biotin immunohistochemical protocol with Ultra Vision Detection System Anti-rabbit and Ultra Vision Detection System ONE (Thermo Fisher Scientific) with diaminobenzidine as the chromogen (Thermo Fisher Scientific Inc., Fremont, CA, USA). Sections were dewaxed, rehydrated, and treated with a 3% solution of H_2O_2 to block endogenous peroxidase. The antibodies to glial acidic protein (GFAP) (ready-to-use, mouse; 1:100, rabbit, Thermo Fisher Scientific), and to neuron-specific beta-3-tubulin (1:100, Abcam) were used for an hour at room temperature as a primary antibody. Negative control sections, in which the primary antibody was omitted, were used for each case in each immunostaining run.

2.3. Morphometry and Statistical Analysis

Five non-overlapping observation fields for each of gecko were selected within five random sections, both in anterior and posterior cerebella, which were stained using Nissl or the antibody to NST. Each field was captured bya Sony digital camera (SSc–Dc50P) mounted on a Leica DM LS light microscope using a 40x objective. On each photomicrograph of the animals, which were cerebellum stained using Nissl, the ratio of the quantity of Purkinje cells with different morphological changes to the total number of Purkinje cells was counted and analysed. In addition, we counted the cells with clearly defined nuclei, demonstrating intense immunoreactivity to NST in comparison with the others cells in the same cerebellar sample, and calculated overstained cells/whole amount of immunoreactive cells. Purkinje cell process (dendrite) density was measured in the anterior and posterior cerebellum for four geckos from the FG and for six geckos from the DSC group.

One hundred and five non-overlapping fields of the molecular layer from the five separate sagittal sections were chosen for each case using the 100x objective (Figure 3d). Each field of interest on the microphotos was 350x350 px. The NST immunopositive dendrite area was calculated as a percentage of total area of the field of interest using ImageJ software tools (the segmentation procedure was performed with the default plugin).

A statistical software package was used (Statistica 6.0, Statsoft Inc., Tulsa, OK, US). Data were compared using the Kruskal-Wallis followed by Mann-Whitney U nonparametric tests to search for differences among all groups and between two groups, respectively. The p-value < 0.05 was considered statistically significant.

3. Thick-Toed Gecko Cerebellum after Long-Term Spaceflight

In general, the histological appearance of the cerebellum was normal in all groups of geckos. In the thick-toed geckos, as in several other groups of lacertilians (Larsell, 1926), the cerebellar layers are everted in comparison with those of other vertebrates (Figure 2a-d). There is one main transverse groove in the thick-toed gecko cerebellum (Figure 2a) and the deep sulcus medianus is clearly visible in the posterior cerebellum (Figure 2b). The granular layer is laminated, which is clearly visible on the sagittal sections (Figure 2a).

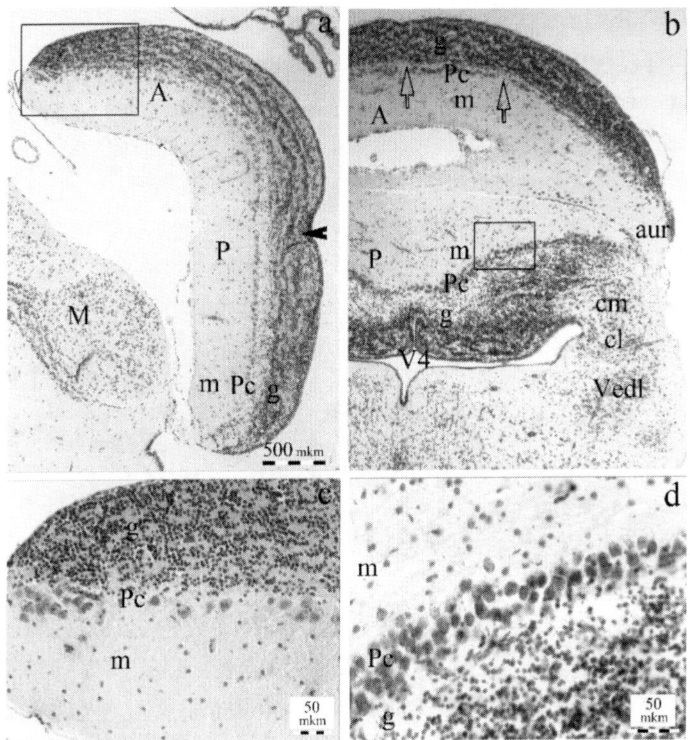

Figure 2. The sagittal (a, c) and coronal (b, d) sections of the DSC thick-toed gecko cerebellum (Nissl staining): a transverse cerebellar groove marked by arrowhead (a), free-Purkije cell longitudinal zones are marked by outlined arrows (b); high-magnifications of zones depicted by frames on a-b correspondingly (c-d): A – anterior cerebellum, aur – auriculi (flocculi) cerebelli, cm, cl – medial and lateral cerebellar nuclei, g – granular cerebellar layer, M – mesencephalon, m – molecular cerebellar layer, P – posterior (basal) cerebellum, Pc – Purkinje cell layer, Vedl – nucleus vestibularis dorsolateralis, V4 – ventriculus quartus.

In the Purkinje cells of the posterior cerebellum of geckos with heterogeneous nonspecific cytomorphological changes (Figure 3a-b), such as chromatolysis (tigrolysis) of different intensity, abnormal vacuolization, and hyperchromatosis, were observed. A significant increase in the number of Purkinje cells with these alterations was revealed in the posterior cerebella of the geckos from the F group in comparison with the control groups. The number of Purkinje cells with signs of hyperchromatosis, chromatolysis, and vacuolization reached an average of 10% in the posterior cerebellum of geckos from the F group, while it was only 4% in control groups (Figure 3e) (Kruskal-Wallis test, $p = 0.016$).

However, some neurons with these changes were also observed in the cerebellum of the geckos from both control groups. No significant differences were detected between the control groups (Proshchina et al., 2017). In our previous study, similar cytological changes were revealed in the neuron somata of vestibular nuclei of rhombencephalon in geckos after the spaceflight on board the Foton-M3 satellite (Russia, 2007, 12 days). These changes are mostly expressed in the large neurons of the ventrolateral vestibular nucleus (*nucleus vestibularis ventrolateralis*), but can also be seen in other nuclei of the vestibular area (*n. vestibularis descendens, n. vestibularis dorsolateralis*) and reticular formation (Proshchina et al., 2008).

Similar data were obtained during the Purkinje cell study using immunohistochemistry with antibodies to NST. In some cells of the vestibular cerebellum of animals from all groups, NST immunoreactivity was heterogeneous (decreasing in some cases and increasing in others) (Figures 3c, 3f) (Proshchina et al., 2017). An increase in the number of Purkinje cells of the posterior cerebellum with an altered reaction to NST in the flight group was revealed during morphometric analysis (average 10% vs 4% in both controls; Kruskal-Wallis test, $p = 0.049$) (Figure 3b).

Heterogeneous nonspecific changes, such as altered NST immunoreactivity, were also observed in the anterior cerebellum in all experimental groups, but we identified no significant differences in the distribution of the cells with aforementioned cytomorphological changes and altered NST immunoreactivity of Purkinje cells in the anterior cerebellum of geckos. Thus, it is reasonable to speculate that the conditions of the spaceflight did not cause hard disturbances of cerebellar proprioception in geckos. Perhaps the reason for this is their ability to preserve almost normal adhesion in weightlessness.

Thus, pathomorphological changes in the Purkinje cells were revealed only in the posterior cerebellum of geckos after a long-term spaceflight.

Such cytomorphological alterations are usually mentioned as primary signs of neurodegenerative changes (Rohkamm, 1977).

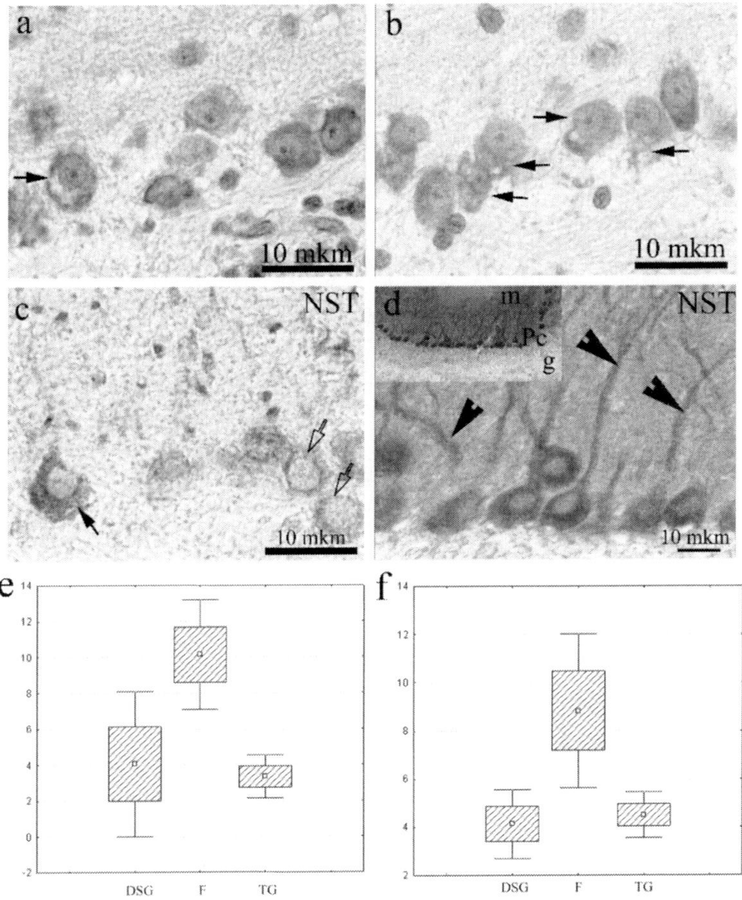

Figure 3. Nissl preparation (a-b) and NST-immunoreactivity on the coronal (a-c) sections of the Purkinje cell layer of geckos from F group: chromatolysis of different intensity (a) and vacuolization (b) marked by arrows; NST-overimmunostaned cell marked by black-arrow and cells with normal NST-immunoreactive intensity – by outlined arrows (c). NST-immunoreactivity in the sagittal section of the Purkinje cell layer: Purkinje cell dendrites are marked by arrowheads (d), low-magnification is inserted. Ratio of the quantity of Purkinje cells with pathomorphological changes (e) and with a changed reaction to NST (f) to the total number of Purkinje cells, provided as the ±mean standard error of the mean ±1.96 standard error of the mean. g – granular cerebellar layer, m – molecular cerebellar layer, Pc – Purkinje cell layer.

However, tinctorial heterogeneity of nerve cells is a nonspecific manifestation of the *in vivo* state of neurons, which correlates with the level of their metabolism (Shantha et al., 1967; Rohkamm, 1977). Hyperchromatosis appears as excessive hyper-staining of Nissl substance (tigroid masses) and evidence of hyperactivity of neurons (Shade and Ford, 1973). Cell swelling, central and segmental chromatolysis increase, and ectopia of the cell nucleus are evidence of functional loading of neurons. Vacuolization first begins from the cytoplasmic periphery and then expands to the whole cell soma, dendrites, and axon. Subtotal and total chromatolysis, vacuolization, and cell swelling (in the case of unimpaired main cell structures) indicate prolonged functional loading on neurons, which only potentially lead to cell injuries, and only pyknosis of nuclei corresponds to neuronal damage (Snesarev, 1950). These neuron features are nonspecific and could be observed in the CNS during different non-pathogenic (short-term functional loading) and pathogenic (local injury, ischemia, toxicosis, long-term stress) conditions. Chromatolysis, abnormal vacuolization, and hyperchromatosis are reversible neuronal changes (Colmant, 1965; Rohkamm, 1977). Thus, we speculate that the aforementioned cytomorphological changes reflect the functional load on the Purkinje cells of the posterior cerebellum. This is evidenced also by the Purkinje cell processes measurements; there were no differences in the Purkinje cell dendrite density of the geckos between F and DSC (average 39.7% and 41.8%, respectively, with individual variation overloading the 2% difference).

Our data coincide with the results of the study on the rat vestibular apparatus. An increase in the number of synapses in the receptor region of the semi-circular canals (Ross, 1994), and the hair cells of the first and second type, which returned to baseline after landing (Ross, 2000), was revealed. It is interesting that the number of synapses of the hair receptors is reduced during hyper-gravity (Lim et al., 1974; Lychakov et al., 1988; Ross, 1993). These data obtained in rats may indicate an increase in functional load on the vestibular apparatus during adaptation to weightlessness. Apparently, the otolith apparatus of the inner ear has mechanisms for adaptation to changes in gravity, as evidenced by changes in the mass of otolith in response to micro- (increase) and hyper-gravity (decrease) from different vertebrates (rats – Vinnikov et al., 1980; Ross et al., 1985; Ross, 1987; Lychakov et al., 1989; Lim et al., 1974; Krasnov, 1991; tadpoles and tritons – Wiederhold et al., 1997; and fish – Wiederhold et al., 2000; Anken et al., 1998). The change in otolith mass is considered to be an adaptation to the changing of gravity to maintain constant pressure on macula (Cohen et al., 2005). On the basis of this anatomical organization, we expect that changes in the linear acceleration stimuli will cause some changes in Purkinje cells. Our data regarding alterations in Purkinje cells coincide with the results of a study of the rat cerebellar cortex after a 24h flight (Holstein et al., 1999) and altered gravity (Bruce, 2003; Krasnov, 1994; Sajdel-Sulkowska et al., 2005). However, in some studies, such results were interpreted as evidence for decreasing vestibular afferentation and, thus, functional activity of the cells (Krasnov, 2008; Krasnov and Krasnikov, 2009). At the same time, in adult mice exposed to very strong vestibular stimuli, the Purkinje neurons in the cerebellum – and perhaps other vestibular neurons as well – respond with morphological changes comparable to those occurring in long-term depression (Bruce, 2003).

In addition, a few small cells scattered in the molecular layer and numerous cells in the granule layer were identified. The neurons in the molecular and granule cerebellar layers demonstrated no difference in distribution between the flight and control groups.

In the molecular layer of the gecko posterior cerebellum, immunoreactivity with GFAP antibodies was observed in the rare astrocytes and numerous processes of cells located around Purkinje cells, which can be attributed to Bergmann glia (Figure 3d). In the current study, we report no differences in the immunoreactivity patterns and intensity of reaction with GFAP antibodies between the F and both control groups. We have previously shown alterations in radial glia in the forebrain cortex of thick-toed geckos after a spaceflight (Proshchina et al., 2008). Immunoreactivity to GFAP antibodies in the medial cortex of geckos after completion of spaceflights on board Foton-M2 and Foton-M3 satellites was lower than in gecko control groups. It is important to note that the duration of these space flights was less than that of "BION-M" No. 1 (16, 12, and 30 days, respectively). Moreover, the animals on both Foton-M2 and Foton-M3 satellites did not eat or drink. It is likely that the differences in our results are connected with the different conditions present during the experiments. According to Uva et al., (2002) cytoskeletal and nuclear changes (micro- and intermediate filament disorganization, derangement of the radial organization of the microtubules, deformity of chromatin condensation, and DNA fragmentation) of the cultured glial cells were also observed in the clinostat study of microgravity effects after 30 min of exposure. However, cytoskeletal reorganization of glial cells and mitotic figures already appeared after 20 h under experimental conditions (Uva et al., 2002). The absence of visible changes in cerebellar glial cells after the spaceflights confirms our assumption about the possibility of a speedy recovery of the Purkinje cells after the alterations emerging under spaceflight conditions, as the increase in the number of astrocytes (astrogliosis) is one of the hallmarks of neurodegenerative disorders (Lukaszevicz et al., 2002). Moreover, changes in Bergmann glia also lead to various disorders in the functioning of Purkinje cells (Riquelme et al., 2002).

All of the described features of the cerebellum after long-term spaceflight may be connected not only with the reversible vestibular system's adaptation to weightlessness, but also with the training of animals to implement motor functions under unusual conditions (Saveliev et al., 2016). The cerebellum is responsible not only for coordination, but also for the formation of new motor skills (Rochefort et al., 2013; Dickson et al., 2016). Sometimes during flotation, the thick-toed geckos were reasonably calm; they could look about, choosing a place to attach. Then, via the bending of their tails and bodies, and, sometimes, rowing motions of their paws, they approached achosen place and attached to it, thereby coordinating their motor activity in weightlessness. Previously, the ability to coordinate motor activity under spaceflight conditions was considered a characteristic only of humans and anamnia. Other animals floated erratically or rotated in conditions of weightlessness (Lychakov, 2015, 2016).

CONCLUSION

Cytomorphological features of cell functional loading (hyper-chromatosis, chromatolysis, and abnormal vacuolization) were observed in the Purkinje cells of the posterior cerebellum of geckos after the spaceflight. These results coincide with the behavioral changes of geckos during the spaceflight. All cytomorphological changes observed in the study were short-term, reversible adaptations. The gecko (*Chondrodactylus turneri* GRAY 1864) is a prospective model to study the vestibular cerebellum of vertebrates in orbital experiments due to the relative simplicity of its organization and, at the same time, its similarities with other vertebrates.

ACKNOWLEDGMENTS

This study was supported by the Russian Foundation for Basic Research (grant № 16-04-00815), the Autonomous Nonprofit Institution "Institute of Biomedical Problems" (ANO IBP) and the Institute of Biomedical Problems (IBMP), the State Scientific Center of the Russian Federation and Federal State Budgetary Institution of Science (Moscow). The project was organized by the Russian Federal Space Agency, the Russian Academy of Sciences, the Russian Space Center "Progress" and the RSCE "Energy." We are very grateful for developing of RSB, creative intellectual and technical collaboration to our colleagues from the St. Petersburg Branch of FSUE "EPM" FMBA Russia - SKTB Biofizpribor.

REFERENCES

[1] Almeida, E. A. C., Roden. C., Phillips, A., Yusuf, R., Globus, R. K., Searby, N., Vercoutere, W., Morey-Holton, E., Gulimova, V., Saveliev, S., Tairbekov, M., Iwaniec, U. T., Mcnamra, A. J., Turner, R. T. Development of the gecko (*Pachydactylus bibronii*) animal

model during Foton m-2 to study comparative effects of microgravity in Terrestrial and aquatic organisms. *J. Gravit. Physiol.* 2006. 13(1), 193-6.

[2] Andreev-Andrievskiy, A., Popova, A., Boyle, R., Alberts, J., Shenkman, B., Vinogradova, O., Dolgov, O., Anokhin, K., Tsvirkun, D., Soldatov, P., Nemirovskaya, T., Ilyin, E., Sychev, V. Mice in Bion-M 1 space mission: training and selection. *PLoS One.* 2014. 9 (8), e104830.

[3] Anken, R. H., Kappel, T., Rahmann, H. Morphometry of fish inner ear otoliths after development at 3 g hypergravity. *Acta Otolaryngol.* 1998. 118 (4), 534–539.

[4] Bangma, G. C., ten Donkelaar, HJ. 1982. Afferent connections of the cerebellum in various types of reptiles. *J. Comp. Neurol.* 207 (3), 255–273.

[5] Bangma, G. C., ten Donkelaar, H. J. Some afferent and efferent connections of the vestibular nuclear complex in the red-eared turtle *Pseudemys scripta* elegans. *J. Comp. Neurol.* 1983 Nov 10;220(4): 453-64.

[6] Bangma, G. C., ten Donkelaar, H. J. Cerebellar efferents in the lizard Varanus exanthematicus. I. Corticonuclear projections. *J. Comp. Neurol.* 1984 Sep 20;228(3):447-59.

[7] Barabanov, V., Gulimova, V., Berdiev, R., Saveliev, S.. Object play in thick-toed geckos during a space experiment. *J. Ethol.* 2015. 33 (2), 109–115.

[8] Barabanov, V. M., Gulimova, V. I., Berdiev, R. K., Saveliev, S. V. Attachment of Turner's thick-toed geckos (*Chondrodactylus turneri* GRAY 1864) during weightlessness and their responses to flotation. *Life Sci. Space Res.* 2018. 18, 21–28.

[9] Barmack, N. H. Central vestibular system: vestibular nuclei and posterior cerebellum. *Brain Res. Bull.* 2003 Jun; 15;60(5-6): 511-41.

[10] Bruce, L. L. Adaptations of the vestibular system to short and long-term exposures to altered gravity. *Adv. Space Res.* 2003. 32 (8), 1533–1539.

[11] Cancedda, R., Liu, Y., Ruggiu, A., Tavella, S., Biticchi, R., Santucci, D., Schwartz, S., Ciparelli, P., Falcetti, G., C., T., Cotronei, V., Pignataro, S., 2012. The mice drawer system (MDS) experiment and the space endurance record-breaking mice. *PLoS One* 7 (5), e32243.

[12] Cohen, B., Yakushin, S. B., Holstein, G. R., Dai, M., Tomko, D. L., Badakva, A. M., Kozlovskaya, I. B. Vestibular experiments in space. *Adv. Space Biol. Med.* 2005. 10, 105–164.

[13] Colmant, H. J., 1965. Zerebrale Hypoxie. in: *Zwanglose Abhandlungen aus dem Gebiet der normalen und pathologischen Anatomie*, Stuttgart: G. Thieme Enke Verlag, Heft 16, 93 p. [Cerebral hypoxia. in: *Casual essays in the field of normal and pathological anatomy*]

[14] Dickson, P. E., Cairns, J., Goldowitz, D., Mittleman, G. Cerebellar contribution to higher and lower order rule learning and cognitive flexibility in mice. *Neuroscience,* 2016. doi: https://doi.org/10.1016/j.neuroscience.2016.03.040.

[15] Goodman, D. C., Simpson, Jt. Jr. Cerebellar stimulation in the unrestrained and unanesthetized alligator. *J. Comp. Neurol.* 1960 Apr; 114:127-35.

[16] Goodman, D. C. The evolution of cerebellar structure and function. *Am. Zool.* 1964 Feb.; 4 (1): 33-36.

[17] Holstein, G. R., Kukielka, E., Martinelli, G. P. Anatomical observations of the rat cerebellar nodulus after 24 hr of spaceflight. *J. Gravit. Physiol.* 1999. 6 (1), 47–50.

[18] Ibsch, M., Anken, R. H., Rahmann, H. Weightlessness during spaceflight results in enhanced synapse formation in a fish brain vestibular nucleus. *Neurosci Lett.* 2000. 296(1), 13-6.

[19] Jamon, M. The development of vestibular system and related functions in mammals: impact of gravity. *Front. Integr. Neurosci.* 2014. 8, 11.

[20] Kalb R., Solomon, D. Space exploration, Mars, and the nervous system. *Arch. Neurol.* 2007. 64(4), 485-90.

[21] Khvatov, I. A., Gulimova, V. I., Barabanov, V. M., Sokolov, A. Yu., Saveliev, S. V., Kharitonov, A. N.. Peculiar features of the adaptive behavior of thick-toed geckos in the orbital spaceflight experiment.

Eksperimental'naya psikhologiya [*Exp Psychol (Russia)*]. 2014. 3, 44–56 (in Russian).

[22] Koppelmans, V., Bloomberg, J. J., Mulavara, A. P., Seidler, R. D. Brain structural plasticity with spaceflight. *NPJ Microgravity*. 2016. 2, 2.

[23] Krasnov, I. B. The otolith apparatus and cerebellar nodulus in rats developed under 2G-gravity. *Phisiologist.* 1991. 34 (1), 206–207 (in Russian).

[24] Krasnov, I. B. Electron microscopy analysis of the structural elements of the vestibular input to nodulus Purkinje's cells in rats exposed to a 9-day spaceflight. *Aviakosm. Ekolog. Med.* 2008. 42 (4), 20–27.

[25] Krasnov, I. B., Krasnikov, G. V. Purkinje's cells in the vestibular and proprioceptive segments of rat's cerebellum following 14-day space flight. *Aviakosm. Ekolog. Med.* 2009. 43 (4), 43–47.

[26] Larsell O. The cerebellum of reptiles. *J. Comp. Neurol.* 1926 Aug.; 41(1):59-94.

[27] Larsell O. The development of the cerebellum in man in relation to its comparative anatomy. *J. Comp. Neurol.* 1947 Oct; 87(2):85-129.

[28] Lazzari, M., Franceschini, V. Glial fibrillary acid protein and vimentin immunoreactivity of astroglial cells in the central nervous system of adult Podarcissicula (Squamata, Lacertidae). *J. Anat.* 2001. 198, 67–75.

[29] Lichtenberg, B. K. Vestibular factors influencing the biomedical support of humans in space. *Acta Astronaut.* 1988. 17(2), 203-6.

[30] Lim, D. J., Stith, J. A., Stockwell, C. W., Oyama, J. Observations on saccules of rats exposed to long-term hypergravity. *Aerosp. Med.* 1974. 45 (7), 705–710.

[31] Lukaszevicz, A. C., Sampaio, N., Guegan, C., Benchoua, A., Couriaud, C., Chevalier, E., Sola, B., Lacombe, P., Onteniente, B. High sensitivity of protoplasmic cortical astroglia to focal ischemia. *J. Cereb. Blood Flow Metab.* 2002. 22, 289–298.

[32] Lychakov, D. V. Behavioural and functional vestibular disorders after space flight. 1. Mammals. *Zh. Evol. Biokhim. Fiziol.* 2015. 51 (6), 393–405 (Russian).

[33] Lychakov, D. V. Behavioural and functional vestibular disorders after space flight. 2. Fishes, amphibians and birds. *Zh. Evol. Biokhim. Fiziol.* 2016. 52 (3), 1–16 (Russian).

[34] Minor, L. B. Physiological principles of vestibular function on earth and in space. *Otolaryngol. Head Neck Surg.* 1998. 118 (Pt. 2 (3)), 5–15.

[35] Mori, S. Disorientation of animals in microgravity. *Nagoya J Med Sci.* 1995. 58(3-4), 71-81.

[36] Nikitin, V. B., Proshchina, A. E., Kharlamova, A. S., Barabanov, V. M., Krivova, J. S., Godovalova, O. S., Savelieva, E. S., Makarov, A. N., Gulimova, V. I., Okshtein, I. L., Naidenko, S. V., Souza, K. A., Almeida, E. A. C., Ilyin, E. A., Saveliev, S. V. Comparative Studies of the Thick-Toed Geckos after the 16 and 12 Days Spaceflight in "Foton-M" Experiments. *J Gravit. Physiol. 2008.* 15(1), 285-8.

[37] Oman, C. M., Cullen, K. E. Brainstem processing of vestibular sensory exafference: implications for motion sickness etiology. *Exp. Brain Res.* 2014. 232 (8), 2483–2492.

[38] Proshchina, A. E., Kharlamova, A. S., Barabanov, V. M., Godovalova, O. S., Gulimova, V. I., Krivova, Y. S., Makarov, A. N., Nikitin, V. B., Savelieva, E. S., Saveliev, S. V. Effect of 12- day spaceflight on brain of thick-toed geckos. *J. Gravit. Physiol.* 2008. 15(1), 297–298.

[39] Proschsina, A., Kharlamova, A., Barabanov, V., Gulimova, V., Saveliev S. Vestibular cerebellum of thick-toed geckos (Chondrodactylus turnery GRAY, 1864) and C57/BL6N mice after the long-term space flight on the biosatellite BION-M1. *J. Chem. Neuroanat.* 2017. 79, 58-65.

[40] Riquelme, R., Miralles, C. P., De Blas, A. L. Bergmann glia GABA(A) receptors concentrate on the glial processes that wrap inhibitory synapses. *J. Neurosci.* 2002. 22 (24), 10720–10730.

[41] Rochefort, C., Lefort, J. M., Rondi-Reig, L. The cerebellum: a new key structure in the navigation system. *Front. Neural Circuits.* 2013. 7, 35.

[42] Rohkamm, R. 1977. Degeneration and Regeneration in Neurons of the Cerebellum, In: *Advances in Anatomy, Embryology and Cell Biology*, vol. 53. Springer-Verlag, Berlin Heidelberg New York, pp. 122.

[43] Ross, M. D., Donovan, K., Chee, O. Otoconial morphology in space-flown rats. *Physiologist.* 1985. 28 (6 Suppl), S219–20.

[44] Ross, M. D. Implications of otoconial changes in microgravity. *Physiologist.* 1987. 30 (1 Suppl), S90–3.

[45] Ross, M. D. Morphological changes in rat vestibular system following weightlessness. *J. Vestib. Res.* 1993. 3 (3), 241–251.

[46] Ross, M. D. A spaceflight study of synaptic plasticity in adult rat vestibular maculas. *Acta Otolaryngol.* Suppl. 1994. 516, 1–14.

[47] Ross, M. D. Changes in ribbon synapses and rough endoplasmic reticulum of rat utricular macular hair cells in weightlessness. *Acta. Otolaryngol.* 2000. 120, 490-499.

[48] Sajdel-Sulkowskaa, E. M., Nguona, K., Sulkowskic, Z. L., ct al. Purkinje cell loss accompanies motor impairment in rats developing at altered gravity. *Neuroreport.* 2005. 16 (18), 2037–2040.

[49] Saveliev, S. V., Gulimova, V. I., Barabanov, V. M., Proschsina, A. E., Kurtova, A. I., Krivova, Y. S., Kharlamova, A. S., Buzmakov, A. V., Zolotov, A. V., Senin R. A., Khlebnikov, A. S., Okshtein, I. L., Asadchikov, V. E. Study of the thick-toed geckos and mice caudal vertebrae. In: Grigoriev M., editor. "*Space research project "BION-M1": medical-biological experiments and studies.* Moscow: SSC RF – IBMP RAS; 2016; P. 298-306 (in Russian).

[50] Shade, J. P., Ford, D. H., 1973. *Basic Neurology: An Introduction to the Structure and Function of the Nervous System*, 2nd revised edition Elsevier, Amsterdam 269 p.

[51] Shantha, T. R., Iijima, K., Bourne, G. H., 1967. Histochemical studies on the cerebellum of squirrel monkey (*Saimiri sciureus*). *Acta. Histochem.* 27 (1), 129–162.

[52] Slenzka K. Neuroplasticity changes during space flight. *Adv. Space Res.* 2003. 31(6), 1595-604.

[53] Snesarev, P. E., 1950. *Theoretical Basis of the Pathological Anatomy of Mental Disease.* Medgiz, Moscow 370 p.

[54] Solomides, P., Moyer, E. L., Talyansky, Y., Choi, S., Gong, C., Globus, R. K., Ronca, A. E. Analysis of adult female mouse (*Mus musculus*) group behavior on the International Space Station (ISS). In: *Annual meeting of the American Society for Gravitational and Space Research* (ASGSR 2016); 32nd; 26–29 Oct. 2016.

[55] Thornton, WE, Bonato, F. Space motion sickness and motion sickness: symptoms and etiology. *Aviat. Space Environ. Med.* 2013. 84(7), 716-21.

[56] Uva, B. M., Masini, M. A., Sturla, M., Prato, P., Passalacqua, M., Giuliani, M., Tagliafierro, G., Strollo, F. Clinorotation-induced weightlessness influences the cytoskeleton of glial cells in culture. *Brain Res.* 2002. 934 (2), 132–139.

[57] Vinnikov, I. A., Lychakov, D. V., Pal'mbakh, L. R., Govardovski ı, V. I., Adanina, V. O. Vestibular apparatus study of the toad, *Xenopus laevis*, and rats under prolonged weightlessness. *Brain Res.* 1980. 934 (2), 132–139.

[58] Von Beckh, H. J. Experiments with animals and human subjects under sub and zero-gravity conditions during the dive and parabolic flight. *J. Aviat. Med.* 1954. 25(3), 235-41.

[59] Voogd, J., Glickstein, M. The anatomy of the cerebellum. *Trends Neurosci.* 1998 Sep; 21(9): 370-5.

[60] Wassersug, R. J., Roberts, L., Gimian, J., Hughes, E., Saunders, R., Devison, D., Woodbury, J., O'Reilly, J. C. The behavioral responses of amphibians and reptiles to microgravity on parabolic flights. *Zoology* (Jena). 2005. 108(2), 107-20.

[61] Wiederhold, M. L., Gao, W. Y., Harrison, J. L., Hejl, R. Development of gravity-sensing organs in altered gravity. *Gravit. Space Biol. Bull.* 1997. 10 (2), 91–96.

[62] Wiederhold, M. L., Harrison, J. L., Parker, K., Nomura, H. Otoliths developed in microgravity. J. *Gravit. Physiol.* 2000. 7 (2), 39–42.

[63] Yamada, K., Watanabe, M. Cytodifferentiation of Bergmann glia and its relationship with Purkinje cells. *Anat. Sci. Int.* 2002. 77 (2), 94–108.

[64] Young, L. R., Oman, C. M., Watt, D. G., Money, K. E., Lichtenberg, B. K. Spatial orientation in weightlessness and readaptation to Earth's gravity. *Science.* 1984. 225, 205–208.

In: Development of the Cerebellum
Editor: Severina Fabbri
ISBN: 978-1-53614-317-1

Chapter 5

Retina Protection with Cerebellum Activation in Experimental Diabetes and Translational Perspectives

Leonid S. Godlevsky[1,*], PhD, Nataliya V. Kresyun[2], PhD, Hanna O. Son[3], MD, Vladlena V. Godovan[3], PhD, Oxana N. Nenova[1], PhD, Mihail P. Pervak[4], MD, Tamara L. Godlevska[5], PhD, Katerina A. Bidnyuk[1], PhD and Tatyana V. Prybolovets[1]

[1]Department of Biophysics, Informatics and Medical Devices, Odesa National Medical University, Odesa, Ukraine
[2]Department of Ophthalmology, Odesa National Medical University, Odesa, Ukraine
[3]Department of General and Clinical Pharmacology, Odesa National Medical University, Odesa, Ukraine
[4]Department of Simulative Medicine, Odesa National Medical University, Odesa, Ukraine
[5]Department of Pediatrics, Odesa National Medical University, Odesa, Ukraine

[*]Corresponding Author Email: godlevskyleonid@yahoo.com.

Abstract

Introduction: Diabetes deteriorates visual pathway functioning, which manifests as a longer viual evoked potential (VEP) latency and reduced wave amplitude. These deteriorations indicate retinopathy development, which is severe and resistant to diabetes treatment. Cerebellar electrical stimulation (ES) does not directly affect VEPs. However, possible curative effects on retinopathy pathogenesis are expected because cerebellar stimulation produces a wide range of positive effects on different brain pathologies.

Methods: The experimental part of the investigation used male Wistar rats with STZ-induced (60.0 mg/kg, i.p.) diabetes. High-frequency (100 Hz) ES was delivered to the VI lobula of the paleocerebellum using two different regimes, with one ES session every two days or thrice ES sessions daily. VEPs were recorded 6 and 12 weeks after diabetes induction. The control groups comprised intact sham-stimulated diabetic rats. VEPs were recorded in patients with newly diagnosed diabetes mellitus after low-intention repeated transcranial magnetic stimulation (rTMS), followed by measurements after sham-rTMS and intensive rTMS.

Results: The latencies of P1, N1, and P2 increased from 18.8% to 22.3% six weeks after STZ-diabetes induction compared to those of control rats. Chronic high-frequency cerebellar ES prevented the elongation of latency in diabetic rats. This preventive effect of ES was pronounced in rats with intensive ES, and it was not followed by body weight or glucose level modifications. Twelve weeks of ES failed to prevent the enlargement of VEP latency.

The P100 latency in patients with diabetes mellitus exceeded those of age-matched controls by 9.6% - 13.5% ($P<0.05$). Photostress after sham stimulation increased the mean VEP latency during the first 20 s, and it did not return to baseline until 60 s of observation. rTMS (1Hz) prevented photostress-induced elongation of the P100 latency, and the mean latency during the post-stress period was not significantly different from that of the control group.

Conclusion: High-frequency ES of the VI lobula of the paleocerebellar cortex in STZ-induced diabetic rats and cerebellar rTMS in patients with newly diagnosed diabetes mellitus improved the diabetes-induced elongation of VEP wave latency.

Keywords: diabetes, streptozotocin, retinopathy, visual-evoked potential, cerebellum, electrical stimulation, transcranial magnetic stimulation, rats, diabetes mellitus

1. INTRODUCTION

Diabetes is a disease with serious systemic complications, such as retinopathy, which is one of the most deteriorative conditions that is resistant to treatment [20, 50, 68]. Diabetes duration affects the development of retinopathy [71], and a history of disease longer than 20 years inevitably precipitates retinopathy with an extremely high risk of blindness.

The pathogenesis of retinopathy involves some common mechanisms of the nervous system and retina. One mechanism is excessive an accumulation of glutamate, which causes neurodegeneration, microglial activation, neoangiogenesis, and oxidative stress [48, 70, 89]. Parkinson's disease (PD) and diabetes retinopathy (DR) exhibit similar leading pathogenic mechanisms [67, 78]. The resemblance between PD and DR is supported by data of subthalamic nucleus deep brain stimulation (DBS) in PD patients, which heightened dopaminergic activity [31, 84]. Color vision was improved, and motor disturbances were alleviated during the course of DBS [19]. Subthalamic DBS prevented retinal thinning in PD patients [54].

Functional improvement of the retina with subthalamic DBS likely results from increased dopaminergic functions because dopamine deficit is one mechanism of retinopathy precipitation [1, 3, 11, 67]. Notably, subthalamic stimulation involves cerebellar structures [36, 57, 77], and the cerebellum activates the dopaminergic system [55] that contributes to PD development [28, 53]. Therefore, these data suggest an intermediate role of cerebellar structures in subthalamic DBS, which may produce the beneficial effects of cerebellar ES on retinopathy. This hypothesis is strengthened by the ability of cerebellar ES to increase adenosine [39, 41, 43] and improve the antioxidant potential in the brain and retina [26, 27]. The insufficiency of adenosine and antioxidant defenses are known mechanisms of diabetes retinopathy development [45,83]. Multispectral therapeutic influences on different brain pathologies, including ischemic retinopathy, result from ES of the nucleus fastigii, which is a powerful source of cerebellar output [18]. These data support investigations of cerebellar influences on the development of DR.

Visual-evoked potentials (VEPs) are one of the most informative criteria of the functional state of visual pathways, and characteristic VEPs are observed for DR. Prolonged VEP latency is observed in STZ-induced diabetes, but amplitude differences are contradictory [10, 63]. VEP may reflect disturbances at different locations in the visual pathway [61], but the contribution of retinopathy is prevalent.

Increases in P100 latency and N75-P100 amplitudes were demonstrated in patients with type I and type II diabetes mellitus [4, 30, 35, 68]. Pattern-reversal VEP responses are deranged in diabetic patients prior to the development of retinopathy, which allows a better prognosis for visual dysfunction. [30]. Data on the role of exposure to intense constant stimulation (i.e., photostress) on the recovery time of P100 in patients with DR are contradictory [7], and increased duration [12, 23, 51, 65, 82] and the absence [12, 47, 86] or shortening [5] of changes are observed.

Studies the effects of cerebellar stimulation on VEP also reported contradictory results, such as the absence of VEP modification during cerebellar ES [22, 79]. These ES studies on cerebellar structures likely involved wider brain networks because of polysynaptic involvement, which may result in postponed long-term modulation of mediator and modulator systems that improve retinal function in experimental and clinical diabetes retinopathy. Cerebellar ES induces metabolic effects that increase the antioxidant potential in brain tissue [26, 27, 45] and produce beneficial effects in a wide scope of most actual brain diseases, including motor (ataxia), cognitive and sensorimotor dysfunction [28, 80].

Repeated transcranial magnetic stimulation (rTMS) of the visual cortex markedly influenced electroretinograms [29], and antidromic influences on the visual system via the oligosynaptical networks [2] are expected following cerebellar stimulation.

The present study investigated the effects of chronic ES of the paleocerebellar cortex on the characteristics of the VEP in rats with STZ-induced diabetes. The effects of cerebellar TMS on the dynamics of photostress restoration in patients with diabetes mellitus were also investigated.

2. METHODS

2.1. Experimental Diabetes

2.1.1. Animals

Wistar male rats, aged 6 to 9 months, were used in this experiment. Animals were group housed in a room at a constant temperature of 23°C, relative humidity of 60%, 12-12-h dark/light cycle, and fed a standard diet with tap water available *ad libitum* in accordance with international laws and policies (EU Council Directive 86/609, OJ L 358, 18/12/1986 P.0001-0028; National Institute of Health Guide for Care and Use of Laboratory Animals, US National Research Council, 1996 P.21-55].

2.1.2. Surgery

Animals were single-housed after surgery [38]. Anesthesia was performed using ketamine (100 mg/kg, i.p., Farmak, Ukraine). The rat head was shaved of fur and cleaned with iodine prior to incision [24].Rats were placed in a stereotaxic device "SEZh-5" (Bohomoletz Institute of Physiology, Kiev, Ukraine) and anesthetized with a 0.5% Novokain solution (Darnitsa, Kiev, Ukraine) infiltration at all pressure points and the site of skin incision. A 2-cm incision was made along the middle sagittal axis, and all soft tissues were removed from the skull surface for implantation of recording and stimulation electrodes. A 1.5-2.0-mm hole for recording and 4.0 mm hole for stimulation electrodes were drilled through the skull using a standard dentistry portable drill (Colt 1, Charkov, Ukraine).

Nichrome monopolar intracortical electrodes for VEP registration were implanted in the visual cortexes (AP= -7.0; L= 3.0; H= 0.5) of both hemispheres, according to the rat brain atlas [66]. The reference electrode was placed at the sagittal line in the nasal bones.

A bipolar stimulating electrode was placed in the cerebellar vermal cortex (AP= -14 from bregma or -5.5 from lambda; H= 2.0; L= 0.1) [66]. The custom-made nichrome electrodes had a diameter of 0.15 mm and an interelectrode distance of 0.25 to 0.30 mm. Electrodes were insulated with 25-μm polyesterimide, except at the tip. Electrodes were fixed on the cranial surface using quick-solidifying dental cement. A 0.9% NaCl solution (5.0 ml at 35°C) was injected i.p. at the end of surgery to prevent dehydration. A potassium salt of penicillin (100,000 IU/kg, i.m. injection) was administered every 12 h for 48 h postoperatively to prevent infection.

Animals recovered for 10 to 14 days after surgery before observations.

2.1.3. Diabetes Modeling

Diabetes was induced using i.p. streptozotocin (STZ) (Sigma Aldrich.ru, Russia) (60 mg/kg, i.p.), which was dissolved in a sodium-citrate buffer solution (pH 4,5). Rats that exhibited glucose levels higher than 300 mg/dL in venous blood one week after STZ administration were included in the study [45]. Glucose levels were determined in a fasted state at 9.00 AM. Rats received insulin injections (0.5-1.0 IU s.c., two to five injections per week) during all periods of observation [45].

2.1.4. Groups and Design of Experiment

Animals were randomly assigned to the following groups 3 days after STZ administration:

- Control group (n= 9) with implanted electrodes without sham stimulation;
- Sham stimulation group (n= 8), with implanted electrodes and received sham ES at the time course as the high stimulated group;
- Low-intensity ES group (n= 7), received one session of ES every second day;
- High-intensity ES group (n=8), received three daily ES sessions.

ES was initiated one week after STZ administration and continued for the entire period before VEP recordings. VEP recording was performed in all groups 6 and 12 weeks after the first STZ administration.

2.1.5. VEP Recording

VEP recording was performed according to a previously described method [88] and as developed by [37, 56]. Animals were anesthetized with ketamine (100 mg/kg, i.p., Pharmak, Ukraine) and adapted to the dark for 10 min. This approach was justified by the short time adaptation to the subsequent light flashes. Body temperature was monitored using rectal thermometry [TPEM-1, FSU] and maintained at 37°C. Tropicamide eyedrops (0.5%) (Pharmac, Ukraine) were given to induce mydriasis.

A custom-made electrode needle was inserted into the tail as the ground. The electrode impedance was maintained below 5 kΩ (MS5209, MasTech, Ukraine). Recordings were performed using Neuropack Four Model MEM – 4104K (Nihon Kohden Corporation, Japan). EEG signals were recorded 200 ms after visual stimuli presentation, and the sample rate was 2 kHz.

Photostimulation was performed using a custom-made flexible panel of 20 white, high-brightness, light-emitting diodes (LEDs) (each of 5 W power) mounted on concave surface with a focal distance 15.0 cm. We tried to place the stimulated eyeball in focus of the emitting device, with coinciding optical lines of the eyeball and the photostimulator.

Stimulation intensity was measured using the lux-meter "Yu-116" (FSU), and data were converted into candles-steradian per m^2 ($cd\text{-}s/m^2$) [42]. Therefore, stimulation intensity was 3.0 log of scotopic units. Photic stimulation was delivered 100 times at a frequency of 0.1 Hz. All procedures were performed under red illumination (λ max = 650 nm). The opposite eye was covered with black tape during EEG recordings.

2.1.6. Electrical Stimulation

ES was performed using the electrical stimulator ESU-2 (universal electrical stimulator, FSU), at a 100-Hz impulse frequency, 0.25-ms monophasic pulse duration, 50-100 mcA intensity, and 4.5-5.0 s of ES duration, which were manually controlled. The intensity of ES was 20% less than the threshold for behavioral reactions (e.g., arrests of on-going locomotor activity). ES stimulations were repeated every 4 minutes, and any behavioral reaction or interruption of locomotor activity as a result of ES was not registered. However, EEG arousal reactions were registered [27]. Sham stimulations were performed via connecting the electrodes to a stimulator without delivery of an electrical current.

2.1.7. Visual Verification of Electrode Position

All experimental animals were euthanized using nembutal (100 mg/kg, i.p., Ceva, France). The location of the electrodes was verified visually after the electrode was gently removed. Electrocoagulation was performed in the area of the electrode placement using the electrode as an anode to apply direct current with an amplitude of 5.0 mA over 30 s. The zone of coagulated tissue served as a visual marker of the placement of the tip of the electrode [75]. The control of the location of stimulation electrodes revealed their presence in the medial part of vermal cortex with their location in merges of the VI lobule, between AP – from -12.5 to -15.0, and the lateral positions were ±1.0 from the midline.

2.2. Patient Characteristics and Clinical Methods

Eighteen practically healthy individuals (mean age 27.1±4.78 years) and 15 people with insulin-dependent diabetes (mean age 26.47±4.64 year) participated in this research. All subjects gave their written consent for the research. All investigations were performed in accordance to the ethical requirements of the commission on ethics at Odesa National Medical University (Animal Care and Ethics Committee, 2008/84).

The following inclusion criteria for diabetes patients were used: newly diagnosed with diabetes, 20-35 years age; duration of disease not more than 3 years; well corrected vision acuity of 7/10 or higher; absence of signs of proliferative retinopathy; absence or subtle neuropathy; absence of eye disease; an unaltered visual field; and preserved cerebellar function on all neurological tests [14]. Criteria for the inclusion in the control group were an intraocular pressure less than 21 mm Hg, preserved acuity of vision, unaltered visual field and the absence of eye diseases or neurological disorders [44].

All tests were performed in a fasting state prior to insulin administration. This state was important because glucose concentration influences neuronal conductance in diabetic patients [34, 82].

2.2.1. VEP Registration

Participants were adapted to a low level of light in a sound-proof room. Adaptation was complete when the pupil diameter was 3 mm. The recommendations of the International Federation of Clinical Neurophysiology (IFCN) and International Society for Clinical Electrophysiology of Vision (ISCEV) were adhered to during VEP registration [61]. Pattern-VEP technology was used to elicit VEPs [61]. A chess pattern with a contrast degree of 75% and mean luminescence of 120 cd/m^2 was used, and contrast reversion was twice per s. The distance between the subject and the center of the screen center was a 15-s acceptance angle for a single pattern unit. Only the right eye was exposed to the light stimuli, and the other eye was covered with a light impenetrable shield during the test session.

The EEG electrodes were placed at Oz (the active electrode) and Fpz (the reference electrode). The ground was fixed on the left arm. The inter-electrode resistance was below 5kΩ. The signal transmission band was limited to 1-100 Hz. The stimulation artifacts were eliminated, and the VEPs were averaged [61]. Two sessions of stimuli exposure were presented, and a minimal 100 responses were averaged for each session after artifact elimination.

Photic stress was induced using a 30-s -long 200 W lamp placed 20 cm from the eyeball. This light obviously enlightened the retina [65]. A control VEP was recorded before photostress based on an average of 50 evoked responses per patient. VEPs were recorded immediately after the photostress exposure, and the responses were averaged every 20 s sequentially until the moment when the resulting response became identical to the basic control record [65]. The time period until the moment of recovery of the VEP characteristics was used as the main dependent variable of the functional state of the retina [44, 65].

2.2.2. Cerebellar rTMS and Investigation Design

Fifteen people with diabetes underwent an active low-intensity and sham rTMS session at a 1-week interval. rTMS was performed using a 10-times higher intense regimen in the next week (Figure 1).

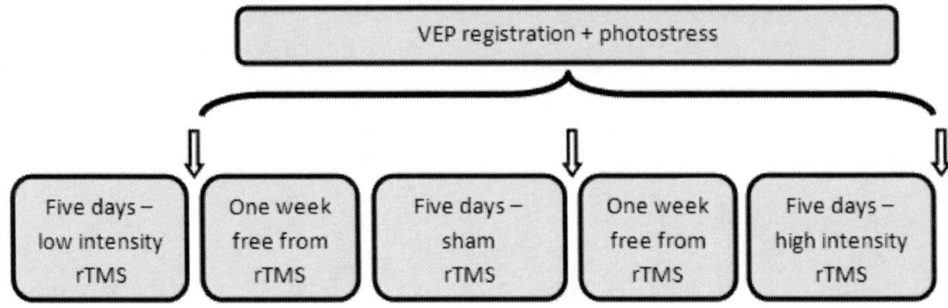

Figure 1. Design of clinical observations of patients with diabetes and cerebellar rTMS.

The Neuro-MS/Ddevice (Neurosoft, Russian Federation) was used for TMS with the appropriate coils, which had a maximal inductivity of 2.0 Tl [44]. The coil was positioned on the middle line of the occipital zone in the tangential plane to the cranium surface according to the adopted cerebellar stimulation technique [21, 52], and the intensive regimen of stimulation included 30 trains of 10-s duration separated by 30-s intervals at 1-Hz frequency [25]. These series of stimulations were performed for five days, and VEP were recorded one hour after the last TMS on the third day. The low-intensity regime of rTMS consisted of three analogous trains delivered for five days. The control group received false stimulation with the coil positioned perpendicularly to the same occipital zone [52].

2.3. Statistical Analysis

VEP latencies and amplitudes were compared using ANOVA and Newman Keuls test. Values are presented as the means ± standard error of the mean (SEM). P values <0.05 were considered significant. Only observations falling between median ± 1.5 SD of the sample were included in the dataset to avoid the influence of outliers. The Shapiro-Wilke's test for normality was used for the latent period.

3. Results and Discussion

3.1. Experimental Data

Weight monitoring revealed that rats with diabetes lost 22.0% of their body weight compared to the starting values (P<0.05) (Table 1). The opposite dynamic of body weight was recorded in the control group (sham-stimulated intact rats), and these animals exceeded their initial weight by 24.0% at 12 weeks (P<0.05). Rats that received the low-intensity stimulation regimen demonstrated a weight loss of 24.9% (P<0.05), and rats with the high intense stimulation lost 22.1% (P<0.05). The concentration of blood glucose was recorded in all groups, and significantly higher values in all groups with STZ diabetes compared to the control group (P's<0.05) (Table 1).

Table 1. Dynamics of body weights and glucose levels in control and diabetic rats with and without cerebellar ES

	Investigated indices	**Before STZ administration**	**6 weeks after STZ**	**12 weeks after STZ**
Control group (n=9)	Body weight in g	259,4±16,2	317,1±27,8	341,2±37,1
	Glucose level in mg/dL	119,3±5,9	113,8±5,31	116,9±5,37
Sham-stimulated rats with diabetes (n=8)	Body weight in g	251,3±15,9	218,3±21,5	196,1±23,9
	Glucose level mg/dL	450,4±33,1	467,1±18,0	420,5± 41,5
One ES per two days (n=7)	Body weight in g	255,7±17,8	211,4±23,1	192,1±25,1
	Glucose level in mg/dL	426,4±37,6	437,0± 43,9	407,5±31,2
Three times daily ES (n=8)	Body weight in g	261,1±16,6	228,9±20,2	203,4±24,3
	Glucose level in mg/dL	435,5±40,2	418,4±35,2	419,6±34,0

3.1.1. 6-Week VEP Measurement

The latencies of P1, N1 and P2 in diabetes sham-stimulated animals exceeded the latencies of the control group by 22.3, 18.8 and 19.8%, respectively (P's<0.05) (Table 2). The VEP indices in rats exposed to the low-intensity ES regimen did not differ from the sham-stimulated diabetes rats (P>0.05). Rats of the intense ES regimen exhibited significantly shorter P1 and N2 latencies compared to the sham-stimulated diabetic rats (by 18.9% and 15.7%, respectively) (P<0.05).

Table 2 shows the characteristics of the VEPs in the four conditions. The amplitude of the P1-N1 was two times lower in diabetic sham-stimulated rats compared to the control group (P<0.05), and the amplitude of the N1-P2 was 43.0% lower (P<0.05). These parameters were continually reduced in the low-intensity ES group, but the reduction in amplitude was not significantly reduced in the high-intensity group compared to the sham group.

Table 2. Characteristics of VEP 6 weeks after STZ administration

	Control (n=9)	**Sham-stimulated diabetes rats (n=8)**	**ES stimulations (one trial in two days) (n=7)**	**ES (three trials daily)(n=8)**
Latency (ms)				
P1	26.77±1.18	34.46±1.65 *	30.64±1.37	27.95±1.26#
N1	43.07±1.95	53.01±2.54*	49.10±2.20	44.71±2.09#
P2	63.29±2.85	78.88±3.82*	73.03±3.37	67.34±3.53
Amplitude (mcV)				
P1-N1	23.56±2.64	12.25±2.36*	11.29±2.15*	19.50±2.73
N1-P2	45.78±6.23	26.13±4.87*	29.14±3.38	33.75±4.14

Notes: *-P<0.05 vs. control group; #-P<0.05 vs. sham stimulated rats with diabetes (ANOVA followed by Kruskall-Wallis test).

3.1.2. 12-Week VEP Measurements

Table 3 present these data. The latencies of P1, N1 and P2 in sham-stimulated diabetes rats exceeded the control rats by 18.0%, 16.3% and 18.5%, respectively (P<0.05). Significant differences in the control group remained present in all diabetes groups (P < 0.05), regardless of weak or intensive stimulation regimens.

Table 3. Characteristics of VEP 12 weeks after STZ administration

	Control (n=9)	**Sham-stimulated diabetes rats (n=8)**	**ES stimulations (one trial in two days) (n=7)**	**ES (three trials daily)(n=8)**
Latency (ms)				
P1	27.62±1.08	33.65±1.56 *	31.70±1.39*	33.80±1.35*
N1	39.64±1.70	47,35+2,3*	45,2+2,21	48,85+2,54*
P2	61.93±2.03	75.98±4.08*	75.63±2.91*	77.10±4.01*
Amplitude (mcV)				
P1-N1	22.75±3.46	11,58+1,92*	10.14±1.77*	13.88±2.76*
N1-P2	42.0±6.60	24.75±3.24*	22.71±3.65*	26.25±3.29*

Note: *-P<0.05 vs. control group; #-P<0.05 vs. sham stimulated rats with diabetes (ANOVA followed with Kruskall-Wallis test).

3.2. Clinical Data

Photostress increased P100 latency in the control group, and the initial value in this group was increased 10.7% (P<0.05) (Table 4).

This effect was recorded during the first 20 s of the post-stress period. The initial P100 latency in all groups with diabetes exceeded the control group by 9.6 - 13.5%. Photostress in sham-stimulated people with diabetes produced a non-significant increase in the P100 latency compared with the initial level. All indices recorded in diabetics after photostress exceeded the control group (P<0.05). The low-intensity rTMS stimulation regimen did not modify post-stress latencies during post-stress sub-periods, and the latency was greater compared to control data, but not different from the diabetes sham-stimulated group.

The latency was 6.2% longer than initial value after intense rTMS (P>0.05) during first 20 s after photostress, which was not different from the control group (P>0.05) (Table 4). Therefore, high-intensity rTMS prevented stress-induced increases in VEP latency.

Table 4. Latency of P100 (in ms) in diabetes patients after cerebellar rTMS

Groups	Before photostress	After photostress (s)		
		20	40	60
Control (n=18)	95.61±10.33	106.95± 10.97#	99.86± 13.83	97.09± 11,27
Diabetes (n=15)	110.57±11.52*	123.91± 19.51*	118.09± 15.11*	114.62± 16,21*
Diabetes + low intensive rTMS (n=15)	108.91±15.60*	120.39±12.59*	115.46±14.23*	112.54+13.63*
Diabetes + intensive rTMS (n=15)	105.72± 12.69*	112.66±11.53	109.01±12.36	105.92± 11.97

Notes: *-P<0,05 vs. control group; #-P<0.05 vs. corresponding value before photostress (ANOVA+Kruskall Wallis test).

Table 5. Amplitude of N75- P100 (in mcV) dynamics in diabetes patients after cerebellar rTMS

Groups	Before photostress	After photostress (s)		
		20	40	60
Control(n=18)	8.79±4.52	6.85± 3.43	7.49± 3.73	8.13± 4.01
Diabetes (n=15)	6.88± 2.21	5.9± 1.96	6.46± 2.37	6.63± 2.03
Diabetes + low intensive rTMS (n=15)	6.69± 1.54	5.87±1.38	5.97±1.66	6.44±1.76
Diabetes + intensive rTMS (n=15)	7.42± 1.90	6.04±1.79	6.88±2.06	7.52± 2.11

The results presented in Table 5 show no clear or significant differences between the four groups with the P75-P100 amplitude before and after photostress (P>0.05).

Our data demonstrated that STZ-induced diabetes in rats and the deterioration of VEP were confined to an increase in latency and reduction in amplitude of wave components. These findings are consistent with the altered VEP characteristics previously described in STZ-induced diabetes models [10, 63, 85]. Chronic high-frequency (100 Hz) ES of cerebellar paleocortex (VI lobula) delivered daily prevented the STZ diabetes-induced increase in VEP latency. Cerebellar stimulations did not affect VEP wave amplitude.

The enlargement of VEP wave latency was recorded six and 12 weeks after STZ administration, but that the preventive effect of ES was found only at week six. This loss of ES effectiveness at later stages of diabetes development may be explained by the intensification of cerebellar morphological deterioration over the developmental time course of experimental diabetes. Notably, glial activation, cellular apoptotic degeneration, and glutamate transport deteriorations develop in the cerebellum of rats with STZ-induced diabetes [33, 60, 62], and these factors may be responsible for the reduced effectiveness of ES.

Our results of cerebellar ES stimulation suggest that the functionality of the cerebellar network was sufficiently preserved at 6 weeks, but deteriorated over the next six weeks. Previous data demonstrated decreased anatomical connections in the cerebellum and cerebro-cerebellar circuits in type II diabetes mellitus patients [20]. Long-lasting diabetes and polyneuropathy produced sensory deficits, pain and temperature sensation disturbances [71], which were followed by difficulties in walking, and stopping automatisms, gait instability and a heightened proneness of falling [50]. This spectrum of symptoms suggests cerebellar involvement in the generation of these pathological manifestations.

These data support a crucial role of preserved cerebellar neuronal networks in the achievement of positive effects of cerebellar stimulation with functional activity of visual pathways. This need for an intact network underlies our inclusion of newly diagnosed diabetes patients without neurological deficit in cerebellar tests. The VEP data in this group demonstrated that the period of recovery of VEP after photostress was prolonged, and this effect was lessened after preliminary trials of cerebellar rTMS. This effect was only observed after intense rTMS was performed daily for five days. Our regimen of cerebellar stimulations is different from previous studies [22, 79], which did not reveal changes in VEP during the period of cerebellar stimulation.

The mechanisms for the preventive effects of cerebellar stimulations with diabetes-induced VEP deteriorations require discussion. Visual inputs to the cerebellum (lobules VI and VII) arise from the superior colliculi via structures in the pons [2, 13, 40]. The cerebellar hemispheres receive visual information from the visual zones of the parietal and temporal cortexes via the pontine nuclei [64]. The involvement of cerebellar structures in visual information perception was estimated using fMRI and revealed activation of vermal lobule VI and right-hemispheric lobule X during the acquisition and discrimination of visual sensory data [8]. A retino-colliculo-cerebellar pathway was identified neurophysiologically [59], and its role was emphasized in avian brain organization [87].

The presence of these oligosynaptic connections support the spreading of antidromic excitation as a consequence of cerebellar ES via these mentioned pathways. This stimulation may activate Muller cells, which are a source of BDNF [72, 73], to initiate the rebuilding of the retinal network. This mechanism may explain the beneficial influence of direct electrical stimulation of the retina [32, 74]. Local stimulation of dopamine and adenosine release [83] as well as retinal vessel dilatation [18, 76] may also be valid. Long-term potentiation (LTP) should also be considered in the excitation spreading effect because long-lasting changes could maintain the influences coming from stimulated cerebellar structures [49].

Prolonged reliable control of hyperglycemia restores the normal characteristics of VEP [34] and abolishes the delay in the restoration of VEP after photostress [82]. Therefore, the contribution of the cerebellum to glucose metabolism and feeding control [6, 9, 16, 69, 90] may also underlie the observed effects of cerebellar stimulation on VEP, despite the lack of effects on body weight and glucose levels in our experimental animals.

Other possible mechanisms of brain stimulations include an influence on genes expression [15, 17, 46, 58]. Profound intrinsic changes in genes activity could produce long-lasting brain stimulation effects and underlies the restriction of neuroinflammation [89], progenitor cell activation and glia response [81].

Conclusion

1) Chronic high-frequency (100 Hz) ES of the paleocerebellum (VI lobula) in rats with STZ-induced diabetes prevented the diabetes-induced enlargement of VEP. This effect was observed at an early stage of diabetes development and was abolished at a later time point.
2) Five days of rTMS (1 Hz, daily) prevented the diabetes-induced retardation of recovery of VEP after photostress in people with newly diagnosed diabetes.

Acknowledgments

We thank Professor Gilles van Luijtelaar for his critical remarks and recommendations.

References

[1] Archibald, N. K., Clarke, M. P., Mosimann, U. P. and Burn, D. J. (2009). The retina in Parkinson's disease. *Brain*, 132(Pt 5): 1128–1145.

[2] Ariel, M. and Fan, T. X. (1993). Electrophysiological evidence for a bisynaptic retinocerebellar pathway.*J Neurophysiol.* 69(4): 1323-1330.

[3] Aung, M. H., Park, H. N., Han, M. K., Obertone, T. S., Abey, J., Aseem, F., Thule P. M., Iuvone P. M. and Pardue, M. T. (2014). Dopamine deficiency contributes to early visual dysfunction in a rodent model of type 1 diabetes. *J Neurosci*, 34(3): 726 DOI: 10.1523/JNEUROSCI.3483-13.2014.

[4] Balta, O., Sungur, G., Yakin, M., Unlu, N., Balta, O. B. and Ornek, F. (2017). Pattern visual evoked potential changes in diabetic patients

without retinopathy. *Hindawi J Ophthalmol,* Article ID 8597629, https://doi.org/10.1155/2017/8597629 .

[5] Baptista, A. M. G., Sousa, R. A. R. C., Rocha, F. A. S. Q., Fernandez, P. S. and Macedo, A. F. (2013). The macular photostress testin diabetes, glaucoma, and cataract *Proceedings of the SPIE*, 8785, id. 8785FW 6 pp.

[6] Batisse-Lignier, M., Rieu, I., Guillet, C., Pujos, E., Morio, B., Lemaire, J. J., Durif, F. and Boirie, Y. (2013). Deep brain stimulation of the subthalamic nucleus regulates postabsorptive glucose metabolism in patients with Parkinson's disease. *J Clin Endocrinol Metab,* 98(6): E1050–E1054.

[7] Bavinger, J. C., Dunbar, G. E., Stem, M. S., Blachley, T. S., Kwark, L., Farsiu, S., Jackson, G. R. and Gardner, T. W. (2016). The effects of diabetic retinopathy and pan-retinal photocoagulation on photoreceptor cell functionas assessed by dark adaptometry. *Invest Ophthalmol Vis Sci*, 57(1): 208-217.

[8] Baumann, O. and Mattingley, J.B. (2010).Scaling of neural responses to visual and auditory motion in the human cerebellum. *J Neurosci,* 30(12): 4489–4495.

[9] Berntson, G. G., Potolicchio, S. J. and Miller, N. E. (1973). Evidence for higher functionsof the cerebellum: eating and grooming elicited by cerebellar stimulation in cats. *Proceed Nat Acad Sci*, 70(9): 2497-2499.

[10] Biessels, G. J., Cristino, N. A., Rutten, G. J.,Hamers, F. P. T., Erkelens, D. W. and Gispen, W. H. (1999). Neurophysiological changes in the central and peripheral nervous system of streptozotocin diabetic rats. Course of development and effects of insulin treatment. *Brain,* 122(Pt 4): 757–768.

[11] Bodis-Wollner, I. (2009). Retinopathy in Parkinson disease. *J Neural. Transm*, 116(11): 1493. https://doi.org/10.1007/s00702-009-0292-z

[12] Boynton, G. E, Stem, M. S., Kwark, L., Jackson, G.R., Farsiu, S. and Gardner, T.W. (2015). Multimodal characterization of proliferative diabetic retinopathy reveals alterations in outer retinal function and structure. *Ophthalmol*, 122(5): 957–967.

[13] Butchel, H. A., Iosif, G., Marchesi, G. F., Provini, L. and Strata, P. (1972). Analysis of the activity in the cerebellar cortex by stimulation of the visual pathways. *Exp Brain Res,* 15(3): 278-288.

[14] *Cerebellum Function Screening*. Available from: https://www.instructables.com/id/Cerebellum-Function-Test/.

[15] Chervyakov, A. V., Chernyavsky, A. Y., Sinitsyn, D. O. and Piradov, M. A. (2015). Possible mechanisms underlying the therapeutic effects of transcranial magnetic stimulation. *Front Hum Neurosci,* 9:303: doi: 10.3389/fnhum.2015.00303.

[16] Chida, K., Iadecola. C. and Reis, D. J. (1989). Global reduction in cerebral blood flow and metabolism elicited from intrinsic neurons of fastigial nucleus. *Brain Res*, 500(1-2): 177–192.

[17] Creed, M. C., Hamani, C. and Nobrega, J. N. (2012) Early gene mapping after deep brain stimulation in a rat model of tardive dyskinesia: Comparison with transient local inactivation. *Eur Neuropsychopharmacol*, 22(7): 506–517.

[18] Ding, A. D., Zhang, H. and Wang, J. M. (2004). [Protective effect of electrical stimulating cerebellar fastigial nucleus on ischemia and reperfusion-injury of rat retina]. *Zhonghua Yan Ke Za Zhi* [Chinese], 40(6): 400-403.

[19] Dumitrascu, O., Kaminski, J., Rutishauser, U., and Tagliati, M. (2015). Subthalamic nuclei deep brain stimulation improves color vision in patients with advanced Parkinson's disease. *Neurology*, 86(16): Supplement P4. 272.

[20] Fang, P., An, J., Tan, X., Zeng, L. L., Shen, H., Qiu, S. and Hu, D. (2017). Changes in the cerebellar and cerebro-cerebellar circuit in type 2 diabetes. *Brain Res Bull*, 130:95–100. DOI: 10.1016/j.brainresbull.2017.01.009.

[21] Farzan, F., Wu, Y., Manor, B., Anastasio, E. M., Lough, M., Novak, V., Greenstein, P. E. and Pascual-Leone, A. (2013). Cerebellar TMS in treatment of a patient with cerebellar ataxia: evidence from clinical, biomechanics and neurophysiological assessments. *Cerebellum*, 12(5): 707–712.

[22] Ferrucci, R., Marceglia, S., Vergari, M., Cogiamanian, F., Mrakic-Sposta, S., Mameli, F., Zago, S., Barbieri, S., and Priori, A. (2008). Cerebellar transcranial direct current stimulation impairs the practice-dependent proficiency increase in working memory. *J Cogn Neurosci,* 20 (9): 1687 – 1697.

[23] Frost-Larsen, K. and Larsen, H. W. (1983). Nyctometry - a new screening method for selection of patients with simple diabetic retinopathy who are at risk of developing proliferative retinopathy. *Acta Ophthalmol (Copenh)*, 61(4): 353–361.

[24] Geiger,B. M., Frank,L. E., Caldera-Siu,A. D. and Pothos,E. N.(2008). Survivable stereotaxic surgery in rodents. *J Vis Exp*, (20), e880, DOI: 10.3791/880 (2008).

[25] Gironelli, A., Kulisevsky, J., Lorenzo, J., Barnbanoj, M., Pascual-Sedano, B. and Otermin, P. (2002). Transcranial magnetic stimulation of the cerebellum in essential tremor. A controlled study. *Arch Neuro,* 59(3): 413-417.

[26] Godlevsky, L. S., Shandra, A. A., Oleinik, A. A., Vastyanov, R. S., Kostyushov, V. V. and Timchishin, O. L. (2002). TNF-alpha in cerebral cortex and cerebellum is affected by amygdalar kindling but not by stimulation of cerebellum. *Polish J Pharmacol,* 54: 655-660.

[27] Godlevsky, L. S.;Muratova, T. N.;Kresyun, N. V. van Luijtelaar, E. L. J. M. and Coenen, A. M. L. (2014). Anxiolytic and antidepressant effects of electric stimulation of the paleocerebellar cortex in pentylenetetrazol kindled rats. *Acta Neur Exp*, 74 (4): 456-464.

[28] Goetz, M., Vesela, M. and Ptacek, R. (2014). Notes on the role of the cerebellum in ADHD. *Austin J Psychiatry Behav Sci,* 1(3): 1013.

[29] Grimanov, R. F. (2004). Changes in bioelectric activity in the human retina after transcranial magnetic stimulation. *Human Physiology* [Russian], 30(1): 40-42.

[30] Gupta, S., Gupta, G. and Deshpande, V. K. (2015). Visual evoked potential changes in patients with diabetes mellitus without retinopathy. *Int J Res Med Sci,* 3(12): 3591-3598.

[31] Hamani, C., Florence, G., Heinsen, H., Plantinga, B. R., Temel, Y., Uludag, K., Alho, E., Teixeira, M. J., Amaro, E. and Fonoff, E. T.

(2017). Subthalamic nucleus deep brain stimulation: basic concepts and novel perspectives. *eNeuro*, 4(5) e0140-17.2017: 1–14, DOI: http://dx.doi.org/10.1523/ENEURO.0140-17.2017.

[32] Henrich-Noack, P., Sergeeva, E. G. and Sabel, B. A. (2017). Non-invasive electrical brain stimulation: from acute to late-stage treatment of central nervous system damage. *Neural Regeneration Res*, 12 (10): 1590-1594.

[33] Hernandez-Fonseca, J. P., Rincon, J., Pedreanez, A., Viera, N., Arcaya, J. L., Carrizo, E. and Mosquera, J. (2009). Structural and ultrastructural analysis of cerebral cortex, cerebellum, and hypothalamus from diabetic rats. *Expl Diabetes Res*, 2009: Article ID 329632, 12 pages doi: 10.1155/2009/329632.

[34] Hernández, O. H., Aguirre-Manzo, L., Monteón, V., Maldonado-Velázquez, R. L. G. (2018). Visual and auditory long-latency brain potentials in patients with type 2 diabetes mellitus. *Int J Advances in Med Sci*, 3(1): 01-08.

[35] Heravian, J., Ehyaei, A., Shoeibi, N., Azimi, A., Ostadi-Moghaddam, H., Yekta, A. A., Khoshsima, M. J. and Esmaily, H. (2017) Pattern visual evoked potentials in patients with type II diabetes mellitus. *J Ophthalmic Vis Res*, 7 (3): 225-230.

[36] Hilker, R., Voges, J., Weisenbach, S., Kalbe, E., Burghaus, L., Ghaemi, M., Lehrke, R., Koulousakis, A., Herholz, K., Sturm, V. and Heiss, W.D. (2003). Subthalamic nucleus stimulation restores glucose metabolism in associative and limbic vortices and in cerebellum: evidence from a FDG-PET study in advanced Parkinson's disease. *J Cerebral Blood Flow & Metabolism,* 24(1): 7–16.

[37] Iwamura, Y., Fujii, Y., and Kamei, C. (2003). The effects of certain H1-antagonists on visual evoked potential in rats. *Brain Res Bull,* 61(4): 393– 398.

[38] Kamakura, R., Kovalainen, M., Leppäluoto, J., Herzig Karl-H., and Mäkelä, K. A. (2016). The effects of group and single housing and automated animal monitoring on urinary corticosterone levels in male C57BL/6 mice. *Physiol Rep,* 4(3): e12703.

[39] Kamikubo, Y, Shimomura, T, Fujita, Y, Tabata, T, Kashiyama, T, Sakurai, T, Fukurotani, K. and Kano, M. J. (2013). Functional cooperation of metabotropic adenosine and glutamate receptors regulates postsynaptic plasticity in the cerebellum. *Neurosci*, 33(47): 18661-18671.

[40] Khamare, B. S. and Combs, C. M. (1975). Duality in retinocerebellar projections in the rabbit. *Exp Neurol*, 48(3): 610-623.

[41] Klyuch, B. P., Dale, N., and Wall, M. J. (2012). Deletion of ecto-5 '-nucleotidase (CD73) reveals direct action potential-dependent adenosine release. *J Neurosci*, 32 (11): 3842–3847.

[42] Kohzaki, K., Vingrys, A. J. and Bui, B. V. (2008). Early inner retinal dysfunction in streptozotocin-induced diabetic rats. *Invest Ophthalmol Vis Sci*, 49(8): 3595-3604.

[43] Kovács Z. and Dobolyi, A. (2013). Anatomical distribution of nucleoside system in the human brain and implications for therapy. In: *Adenosine: A Key Link between Metabolism and Brain Activity* (Masino S, and Boison D (eds.), Springer Science+Business Media, New York, 621-656.

[44] Kresyun, N. V. (2014). Functional recovery of retina after photostress is accelerated by transcranial cerebellar stimulation in patients with diabetic retinopathy. *Curierul Medical* [Moldova], 57 (1): 13-17.

[45] Kresyun, N. V. and Godlevsky, L. S. (2014). [Superoxiddismutase and catalase activity in the experimental diabetes retina under conditions of paleocerebellar cortex electrical stimulation]. *Bull Exp Biol Med* [Rusian], 158(8): 168-171.

[46] Ljubisavljevic, M. R., Javid, A., Oommen J., Parekh, K., Nagelkerke, N., Shehab, S. and Adrian, T. E. (2015). The effects of different repetitive transcranial magnetic stimulation (rTMS) protocols on cortical gene expression in a rat model of cerebral ischemic-reperfusion injury. *PLoS ONE*, 10 (10): e0139892. doi: 10.1371/ journal.pone.0139892.

[47] Loughman, J., Ratzlaff, M., Foerg, B. and Connell, P. (2014). Suitability and repeatability of a photostress recovery test device, the

macular degeneration detector (MDD-2), for diabetes and diabetic retinopathy assessment. *Retina*, 34(5): 1006-1013.

[48] Lu, L., Jiang, Y., Jaganathan, R. and Hao, Y. (2018). Current advances in pharmacotherapy and technology for diabetic retinopathy: a systematic review. *J Ophthalmol*, 2018: Article ID 1694187, 13 pages, 2018. https://doi.org/10.1155/2018/1694187.

[49] McIntyre, C. C., Savasta, M., Goff, L. K. L. and Vitek, J. L. (2004). Uncovering the mechanism(s) of action of deep brain stimulation: activation, inhibition, or both. *Clin Neurophysiol*, 115(6):1239–1248.

[50] Meier, M. R., Desrosiers, J., Bourassa, P. and Blaszczyk, J. (2001). Effect of type II diabetic peripheral neuropathy on gait termination in the elderly. *Diabetologia,* 44(5): 585-592.

[51] Midena, E., Segato, T., Giuliano, M. and Zucchetto, M. (1990). Macular recovery function (nyctometry) in diabetics without and with early retinopathy. *Br J Ophthalmol*, 74(2): 106–108.

[52] Minks, E., Kopickova, M., Marecek, R., Streitova, H. and Bares, M. (2010). Transcranial magnetic stimulation of the cerebellum. *Biomed Pap Med Fac Univ Palacky Olomouc Czech Repub*, 154(2): 133-139.

[53] Mirdamadi, J. L. (2016). Cerebellar role in Parkinson's disease. *J Neurophysiol*, 116(3):917-919.

[54] Miri, S., Glazman, S. and Bodis-Wollner, I. (2016). OCT and Parkinson disease. In: Grzybowski A. and Barboni P., (Eds.), *OCT in Central Nervous System Diseases: The Eye as a Window to the Brain.* (105-121). Switzerland: Springer International Publishing. DOI: 10.1007/978-3-319-24085-5.

[55] Mittleman, G., Goldowitz, D., Heck, D. H. and Blaha, C. D. (2008). Cerebellar modulation of frontal cortex dopamine efflux in mice: relevance to autism and schizophrenia. *Synapse*, 62(7): 544-550.

[56] Miyake, K. I., Yoshida, M., Inoue, Y. and Hata, Y. (2007). Neuroprotective effect of transcorneal electrical stimulation on the acute phase of optic nerve injury. *Invest Ophthalmol Vis Sci,* 48(5): 2356–2361.

[57] Moers-Hornikx,V. M., Vles, J. S., Tan, S. K., Cox, K., Hoogland, G, Steinbusch, W. M. and Temel, Y. (2011). Cerebellar nuclei are

activated by high-frequency stimulation of the subthalamic nucleus. *Neurosci Lett,*496 (2):111-115.

[58] Mohammadi, A., and Mehdizadeh, A. R. (2016). Deep brain stimulation and gene expression alterations in Parkinson's disease. *J Biomed Phys Eng*, 6 (2): 47-49.

[59] Muroga, T. (1975). Electrophysiological study on colliculocerebellar pathway in cat. *Nagoya J Med Sci*, 38 (1-2): 11-23.

[60] Nagayach, A., Patro, N. and Patro, I. (2014). Experimentally induced diabetes causes glial activation, glutamate toxicity and cellular damage leading to changes in motor function. *Front Cell Neurosci*, 8: 355. doi: 10.3389/fncel.2014.00355.

[61] Odom J. V., Bach, M., Brigell, M., Holder, G. E., McCulloch, D.L. and Tormene, A. P. (2010). ISCEV standard for clinical visual evoked potentials (2009 update). *Doc Ophthalmol*, 120 (1): 111–119.

[62] Ozdemir, N. G., Akbas, F., Kotil, T. and Yilmaz, A. (2016). Analysis of diabetes-related cerebellar changes in streptozotocin-induced diabetic rats. *Turk J Med Sci*, 46(5): 1579-1592.

[63] Ozkaya, Y. G., Agar, A., Haglioglu, G. and Yargicoglu, P. (2007). Exercise improves visual deficit by visual evoked potentials in streptozotocin – induced diabetic rats. *Tohoku J Exp Med*, 213(4): 313-321.

[64] Palesi, F., De Rinaldis, A., Castellazzi, G., Calamante, F., Muhlert, N., Chard, D., Tournier, J. D., Magenes, G., D'Angelo, E. and Gandini Wheeler-Kingshott, C. A. M. (2017). Contralateral cortico-pontocerebellar pathways reconstruction in humans *in vivo*: implications for reciprocal cerebro-cerebellar structural connectivity in motor and non-motor areas. *Sceintific Reports*, (7): 12841 DOI: 10.1038/s41598-017-13079-82.

[65] Parisi, V. and Uccioli, L. (2011). Visual electrophysiological responses in persons with type 1 diabetes. *Diabetes Metab Res Rev,* 17(1): 12-18.

[66] Paxinos, G. and Watson, C. (1998). *The Rat brain in stereotaxic coordinates,* Sydney, Academic Press Inc.

[67] Polo, V., Satue, M., Rodrigo, M. J., Otin, S., Alarcia, R., Bambo, M. P, Fuertes, M. I, Larrosa, J. M., Pablo, L. E. and Garcia-Martin, E. (2016). Visual dysfunction and its correlation with retinal changes in patients with Parkinson's disease: an observational cross-sectional study. *BMJ Open*, 6: e009658. doi: 10.1136/bmjopen-2015-009658.

[68] Pescosolido, N., Barbato, A., Stefanucci, A. and Buomprisco, G. (2015). Role of electrophysiology in the early diagnosis and follow-up of diabetic retinopathy. *J Diabetes Res*, 2015: Article ID 319692, 8 pages http://dx.doi.org/10.1155/2015/319692.

[69] Reis, D. J., Feinstein, D., Galea, E. and Golanov, E. V. (1997) Central neurogenic neuroprotection: protection of brain from focal ischemia by cerebellar stimulation. *Fundam Clin Pharmacol*, 1:I(Suppl1): 39s-43s.

[70] Rubsam, A., Parikh, S. and Fort, P.E. (2018). Role of inflammation in diabetic retinopathy. *Int J Mol Sci*, 19: 942; doi: 10.3390/ijms1904 0942.

[71] Said, G., Baudoin, D. and Toyooka, K. (2008). Sensory loss, pains, motor deficit and axonal regeneration in length-dependent diabetic polyneuropathy. *J Neurol*, 255 (11): 1693-702.

[72] Sato, T, Fujikado, T, Lee, T. S. and Tano, Y. (2008). Direct effect of electrical stimulation on induction of brain-derived neurotrophic factor from cultured retinal Muller cells. *Invest Ophthalmol Vis Sci*, 49(10): 4641-4646.

[73] Sato, T., Fujikado, T., Morimoto, T., Matsushita, K., Harada T. and Tano, Y. (2008). Effect of electrical stimulation on IGF-1 transcription by L-type calcium channels in cultured retinal Muller cells. *Jpn J Ophthalmol*, 52(3): 217-223.

[74] Sehic, A., Guo, S., Cho, K.-S., Corraya, R. M., Chen, D. F. and Utheim, T. P. (2016). Electrical stimulation as a means for improving vision. *Am J Pathology*, 186 (11): 2783-2797.

[75] Shandra, A. A. and Godlevsky, L. S. (2005). Pentylenetetrazol-induced kindling as a model of absence and convulsive forms of epilepsy. In: Corcoran M.E. and Moshe S.L. (Eds.), *Kindling 6*. (49-59). New York: Spinger.

[76] Strohmaier, C. A, Motloch, K., Runge, C., Trost, A., Boqner, B., Kaser-Eichberger, A., Schrödl, F., Lenzhofer, M. and Reitsamer, H. A. (2016). Retinal vessel diameter responses to central electrical stimulation in the rat: effect of nitric oxide synthase inhibition. *Invest Ophthalmol Vis Sci,* 57(11): 4553–4557.

[77] Sutton, A. C., O'Connor, K. A., Pilitsis J. G. and Shin, D. S. (2015). Stimulation of the subthalamic nucleus engages the cerebellum for motor function in parkinsonian rats. *Brain Struct. Funct,* 220 (6): 3595-609.

[78] Tian, T., Li, Z. and Lu, H. (2015). Common pathophysiology affecting diabetic retinopathy and Parkinson's disease. *Med. Hypothesis*, 85(4): 397-398.

[79] Upton, A. R.M. and Cooper, I. S. (1976). Some neurophysiological effects of cerebellar stimulation in man. *Le Journal Canadien Des Sciences Neurologiques*, 3, (4): 237-254.

[80] van Dun, K. and Manto, M. (2017). Non-invasive cerebellar stimulation: moving towards clinical applications for cerebellar and extra-cerebellar disorders. *The Cerebellum*, https://doi.org/10.1007/s12311-017-0908-z.

[81] Vedam-Mai, V., Baradaran-Shoraka, M., Reynolds, B. A. and Okun, M.S. (2016). Tissue Response to deep brain stimulation and microlesion: a comparative study. *Neuromodulation*, 19(5): 451–458.

[82] Verrotti, A., Lobefalo, L., Trotta, D., Loggia, G. D., Chiarelli, F., Luigi, C., Morgese, G. and Gallenga, P. (2000). Visual evoked potentials in young persons with newly diagnosed diabetes: a long-term follow-up. *Developmental Med Child Neurol,* 42(4): 240–244.

[83] Vindeirinho, J., Santiago, A. R., Cavadas, C., Ambrosio, A. F. and Santos, P. F. (2016). The adenosinergic system in diabetic retinopathy. *J Diabetes Res,* Article ID 4270301, 8 pages http://dx.doi.org/10.1155/2016/4270301.

[84] Wang, J., Ma, Y., Huang, Z., Sun, B., Guan, Y. and Zuo, C. (2010). Modulation of metabolic brain function by bilateral subthalamic nucleus stimulation in the treatment of Parkinson disease. *J Neurol*, 25 (7): 72-78.

[85] Wolff, B. E., Bearse Jr., M. A., Schneck, M. E., Barez, S. and Adams, A. J. (2010) Multifocal VEP (mfVEP) reveals abnormal neuronal delays in diabetes. *Documenta Ophthalmologica*, 121 (3): 189–196.

[86] Wu, G., Weiter, J. J., Santos, S., Ginsburg, L. and Villalobos, R. (1990). The macular photostress test in diabetic retinopathy and age-related macular degeneration. *Arch Ophthalmol*, 108(11): 1556–1558.

[87] Wylie, D. R., Gutierrez-Ibanez, C., Gaede, A. H., Altshuler, D. L. and Iwaniuk, A. N. (2018). Visual-cerebellar pathways and their roles in the control of avian flight. *Front Neurosci*, 12: 223. doi: 10.3389/fnins.2018.00223.

[88] You, Y., Klistorner, A., Thie, J. and Graham, S. L. (2011). Latency delay of visual evoked potential is a real measurement of demyelination in a rat model of optic neuritis, *Invest Ophthalmol Vis Sci,* 52 (9): 6911-6918.

[89] Yu, Y., Chen, H. and Su, S. B. (2015). Neuroinflammatory responses in diabetic retinopathy. *J Neuroinflammation*, 12:141, DOI 10.1186/s12974-015-0368-7.

[90] Zhu J. N. and Wang, J. J. (2008). The cerebellum in feeding control: possible function and mechanism. *Cell Mol Neurobiol*, 28(4): 469–478 DOI 10.1007/s10571-007-9236-z.

In: Development of the Cerebellum
Editor: Severina Fabbri

ISBN: 978-1-53614-317-1

Chapter 6

THE (SURPRISING) ROLE OF THE CEREBELLUM IN COGNITIVE FUNCTIONS IN OLD ADULTS

Daniela Aisenberg*[*], *PhD
Department of Clinical Psychology - Gerontology,
Ruppin Academic Center, Emek Hefer, Israel

ABSTRACT

High cognitive abilities were commonly related to the prefrontal cortex. However, in recent years, the cerebellum was found to be strongly associated with age-related decline in motor and executive functions, even beyond the prefrontal cortex.

Theoretical frameworks were suggested to understand the role of the cerebellum: as important for the formation of internal models of behaviour, as important for the timing of behaviour, or as crucial in sequence processing.

Imaging research support the idea that age-related changes in cerebellar activation lead to slowed updating of stimulus-response mapping.

[*] Corresponding Author Email Danielaa@ruppin.ac.il.

Here, a meta-analysis of recent findings of cerebellar involvement in executive functions is provided. Also, a methodological issue is raised, relevant for models explaining cerebellar connectivity and effects on cognitive performance in old age.

The surprising role of the cerebellum, hence, should no longer be surprising, and research of cognitive decline in old adults should take it under consideration.

Keywords: aging, cognitive functions, cerebellum, executive functions, motor tasks

INTRODUCTION

In this chapter I'll review cognitive changes affected by age and show a meta-analysis of findings correlating cerebellar activation to executive functions in old adults. I'll also discuss the common explanations for the surprising role of the cerebellum in age-related cognitive decline, and argue that a methodological issue may still account for these findings, and should be taken under consideration in theoretical interpretation.

COGNITIVE CHANGES WITH AGING

Changes in psychomotor and cognitive performance occur in aging (Craik & Salthouse, 2011). According to Salthouse (2016) this explains deficiencies in the ability to carry out complex activities in old adults.

Age-related effects on cognitive functions were found in various brain networks. Perceptual and motor functions affected by age are reflected in slower performance and reaction time (Craik & Bialystok, 2006). Executive functions were also found to be affected by aging (Grady, 2012), particularly cognitive control and conflict monitoring—the ability to suppress irrelevant information and engage selective attention (e.g., Van Veen & Carter, 2006; Aisenberg, Sapir, Close, Henik & d'Avossa, 2018). At the same time, several domains are found to be differentially affected by aging. For example, semantic memory performance is preserved in healthy old adults, while working memory performance shows age-related decline (Raz et al., 2005; West & Alain, 2000).

CEREBELLUM RELATIONS TO COGNITIVE ABILITIES

In young adults, investigations of the cerebellum showed involvement in various tasks, related to executive functions (Schweizer, Alexander, Cusimano & Stuss, 2007; Schweizer, Oriet, Meiran, Alexander, Cusimano & Stuss, 2007). Correlation of the cerebellum with the pre-frontal cortex was excessively found (Ramnani, 2006). Bischoff-Grethe, Ivry, and Grafton (2002) assessed the effect of specific attentional switching and stimulus-response remapping on the BOLD signal. Right anterior cerebellum activations were associated with response reassignment. The authors concluded that cerebellar activations reflect the updating of stimulus–response associations. Engagement of the cerebellum during stimulus-response reassignment has been confirmed by later studies (Berger et al., 2005). Children who had undergone resections for cerebellar tumors, showed diminished detection accuracy following a cue instructing a change in the task relevant dimension, supporting the involvement of the cerebellum in updating the stimulus response mapping. Interestingly, this impairment was only evident when the cue-target interval was less than 2.5s, suggesting that the cerebellar lesion specifically impaired the ability to rapidly complete the updating (Courchesne et al., 1994).

In old age, impaired motor and cognitive performance was suggested to reflect diminished cerebellar function (Bernard & Seidler, 2014). Specifically, it was argued that the anterior lobe of the cerebellum is particularly vulnerable to aging (Andersen, Gundersen & Pakkenberg, 2003). Executive functions were related to cerebellar volume, particularly the vermis region was correlated with processing speed, memory, and visual reproduction (Miller et al., 2013; Sokunbi et al., 2011; Hogan et al., 2011). Bernard and Seidler, (2013) found positive associations for the posterior cerebellum in working memory, and negative associations in motor performance such as RT and balance. Some studies reported findings regarding the cerebellum but not as part of their focus of attention, and therefore, data is lacking. Several studies did report specific data regarding cerebellum statistics, and these are entered into a statistic meta-analysis, as seen in Figure 1.

In a recent study, we proposed that age related changes in cerebellar activation lead to slowed updating of stimulus response mapping, and thus, loss of sequential effects in the Simon task. Age differences in sequential dependencies were found in the right anterior cerebellum, a region presumably related to sensori-motor transformations (Imamizu, Kuroda, Yoshioka & Kawato, 2004). While young adults showed greater activation in this region in switch trials, that is, when the current and previous target congruency differed, old adults showed greater activation following incongruent targets, regardless of the preceding target congruency. This neural correlate of the aging deficit was compatible to the behavioral pattern, also found in Aisenberg, Sapir, d'Avossa and Henik (2014). We then suggested that in young adults, processes are recruited following each target, which change stimulus-response contingencies, while in older adults this trial to trial updating is impaired. In older adults, this leads to congruency effects that do not change with trial history, both behaviorally and neurologically. This is in line with findings from Molinari and Leggio, (2013).

Another study which expected to find cognitive correlations to pre-frontal regions was conducted by Lee et al. (2005). They examined the relationships between intelligence, using the Weschler adult intelligence scale (WAIS), and gray matter (presumably in the prefrontal cortex). Surprisingly, they did not find correlations with prefrontal cortex, but rather with the posterior cerebellum (but see also Raz, Schmiedek, Rodrigue, Kennedy, Lindenberger & Lövdén, 2013, who found correlations only with the cerebellum, but no correlations of cognitive performance or change due to training with cerebellum volume).

Cognitive functions and the Cerebellum in old age -- $k = 8$ $N = 438$

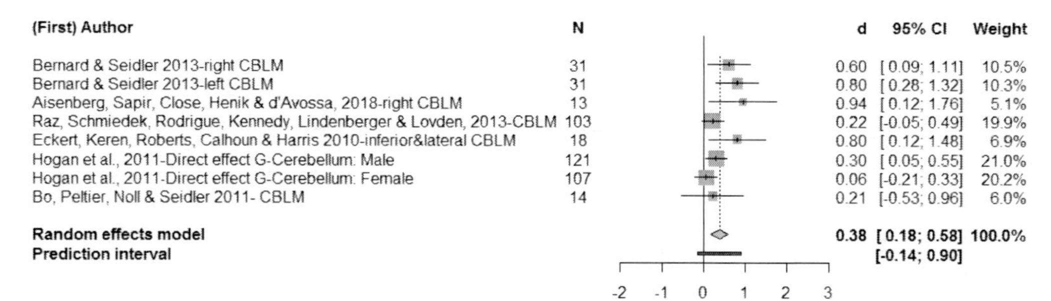

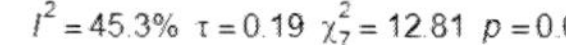

Figure 1. Meta-analysis plot for reported correlations between cognitive functions and cerebellar activation change in old adults. Out of 6,620 results searching Google Scholar for paper dealing with cerebellum/cerebellar cognitive age/aging in the past 10 years, eliminating reviews (120), most papers did not mention the cerebellum specifically in their results. 12 papers matched the criteria for this meta-analysis. Eventually, 6 papers provided relevant data of correlations between cerebellum and specific cognitive functions.

Is It Really the Cerebellum?

Paul et al. (2009), who investigated cognitive functions correlated to cerebellum (vermis) and the prefrontal cortex volume in old adults, found that when controlling for the prefrontal cortex in the analysis of the vermis, the correlations were no longer significant. They suggested that interactions between the cerebellum and cortical regions should be considered. Here I emphasize another consideration. It is important to note, that all studies reported above have used tasks that require (fully or partially) motor skills for successful performance.

Recent studies go back to connecting learning and movement, learning and motor control. Daniel Algom (2003) wrote that after a century of disconnection between sensation and inteligence, research nowadays goes back to the understanding that these domains are related. In other words, understanding high cognitive functions should consider relations to sensory-motor abilities. Indeed, the cerebellum is recognized as supporting associative learning, goal-directed behavior and action execution (Ito, 2006; Giovannucci et al., 2017). In old adults, Bo et al., (2011) recently demonstrated that older adults show less cerebellar activation compared to young adults during symbolic motor learning.

Bernard and Siedler (2014) concluded that "If in advanced age, the cerebellum is further unable to communicate with the cerebral cortex due to degraded connections, important updates about performance due to monitoring of the actual behavior … cannot be transmitted as effectively, resulting in behavioral deficits." (pp. 17). I suggest that perhaps the connection is through the chosen tasks in our research. That is, since we (all) use motor tasks (even for mental performance sometimes), we observe age-related cognitive decline in the cerebellum.

Another explanation was given that goal-directed behavior occurs through connectivity between cerebellum and basal ganglia. Again, I argue that we need to take under consideration the chosen task used to explore this question. Is goal-directed behavior a process involving the cerebellum, or is it the use of a motor task that creates the involvement?

Stoodley (2012) argued that the cerebellum is involved even when motor demands are absent. Balsters, Whelan, Robertson and Ramnani (2012) also showed that the cerebellum can contribute to cognitive control independent of motor control, using abstract stimuli in their study. I believe such differentiation is not necessarely present, specifically according to their agreement that the cerebellum can be broadly divided into functional regions and has wide connectivity between its different regions, and sensory-motor/association areas of the cortex (Stoodley, 2012).

It is clear today that when looking at the formation of internal models of behaviour, timing of behaviour, and sequence processing, the cerebellum has an important role, no longer surprising. As such, in old age, cerebellar changes influence high cognitive processess and contribute to age-related decline. Raz et al., (2013) found that the cerebellum was the only region in which significantly reduced shrinkage was apparent after completion of cognitive training. That provides strong evidence for future work on relevant interventions for improving cognitive abilities and preventing decline in old age.

ACKNOWLEDGMENTS

I wish to thank Avi Kluger for his help in analyzing the data.

REFERENCES

Aisenberg, D., Sapir, A., Close, A., Henik, A. & d'Avossa, G. (2018). Right anterior cerebellum BOLD responses reflect age related changes in Simon task sequential effects. *Neuropsychologia*, *109*, 155-164.

Aisenberg, D., Sapir, A., d'Avossa, G. & Henik, A. (2014). Long trial durations normalise the interference effect and sequential updating during healthy aging. *Acta psychologica*, *153*, 169-178.

Algom, D. (2003). Aging of the senses and its functional implications. In Arnold Rozin (Ed.), *Aging and old age in Israel* (pp. 385-408). Jerusalem: Grafit Ltd.

Andersen, B. B., Gundersen, H. J. G. & Pakkenberg, B. (2003). Aging of the human cerebellum: a stereological study. *Journal of Comparative Neurology*, *466*(3), 356-365.

Balsters, J. H., Whelan, C. D., Robertson, I. H. & Ramnani, N. (2012). Cerebellum and cognition: evidence for the encoding of higher order rules. *Cerebral Cortex*, *23*(6), 1433-1443.

Berger, A., Sadeh, M., Tzur, G., Shuper, A., Kornreich, L., Inbar, D., ... & Kessler, Y. (2005). Task switching after cerebellar damage. *Neuropsychology*, *19*(3), 362.

Bernard, J. A. & Seidler, R. D. (2013). Relationships between regional cerebellar volume and sensorimotor and cognitive function in young and older adults. *The Cerebellum*, *12*(5), 721-737.

Bernard, J. A. & Seidler, R. D. (2014). Moving forward: age effects on the cerebellum underlie cognitive and motor declines. *Neuroscience & Biobehavioral Reviews*, *42*, 193-207.

Bischoff-Grethe, A., Ivry, R. B. & Grafton, S. T. (2002). Cerebellar involvement in response reassignment rather than attention. *Journal of Neuroscience*, *22*(2), 546-553.

Bo, J., Peltier, S. J., Noll, D. C. & Seidler, R. D. (2011). Age differences in symbolic representations of motor sequence learning. *Neurosci Lett.*, *504*, 68–72.

Courchesne, E., Townsend, J., Akshoomoff, N. A., Saitoh, O., Yeung-Courchesne, R., Lincoln, A. J., ... & Lau, L. (1994). Impairment in shifting attention in autistic and cerebellar patients. *Behavioral neuroscience*, *108*(5), 848.

Craik, F. I. M. & Bialystok, E. (2006). Cognition through the lifespan: Mechanisms of change. *Trends in Cognitive Sciences*, *10*, 131-138.

Craik, F. I. & Salthouse, T. A. (Eds.). (2011). *The handbook of aging and cognition*. Psychology Press.

Eckert, M. A., Keren, N. I., Roberts, D. R., Calhoun, V. D. & Harris, K. C. (2010). Age-related changes in processing speed: unique contributions of cerebellar and prefrontal cortex. *Frontiers in Human Neuroscience*, *4*, 10.

Giovannucci, A., Badura, A., Deverett, B., Najafi, F., Pereira, T. D., Gao, Z., ... & De Zeeuw, C. I. (2017). Cerebellar granule cells acquire a widespread predictive feedback signal during motor learning. *Nature neuroscience*, *20*(5), 727.

Grady, C. (2012). The cognitive neuroscience of ageing. *Nature Reviews Neuroscience*, *13*(7), 491.

Hogan, M. J., Staff, R. T., Bunting, B., Murray, A. D., Ahearn, T. S., Deary, I. J. & Whalley, L. J. (2011). Cerebellar brain volume accounts for variance in cognitive performance in older adults. *Cortex; a journal devoted to the study of the nervous system and behavior*, *474*, 441-50.

Imamizu, H., Kuroda, T., Yoshioka, T., & Kawato, M. (2004). Functional magnetic resonance imaging examination of two modular architectures for switching multiple internal models. *Journal of Neuroscience*, *24*(5), 1173-1181.

Ito, M. (2006). Cerebellar circuitry as a neuronal machine. *Prog. Neurobiol.*, *78*, 272–303.

Salthouse, T. A. (2016). *Theoretical perspectives on cognitive aging*. Psychology Press.

Lee, J. Y., Lyoo, I. K., Kim, S. U., Jang, H. S., Lee, D. W., Jeon, H. J., ... & Cho, M. J. (2005). Intellect declines in healthy elderly subjects and cerebellum. *Psychiatry and clinical neurosciences*, *59*(1), 45-51.

Miller, T. D., Ferguson, K. J., Reid, L. M., Wardlaw, J. M., Starr, J. M., Seckl, J. R., ... & MacLullich, A. M. (2013). Cerebellar vermis size and cognitive ability in community-dwelling elderly men. *The Cerebellum*, *12*(1), 68-73.

Molinari, M. & Leggio, M. G. (2013). Cerebellar sequencing for cognitive processing. In *Handbook of the cerebellum and cerebellar disorders* (pp. 1701-1715). Springer Netherlands.

Paul, R., Grieve, S. M., Chaudary, B., Gordon, N., Lawrence, J., Cooper, N., ... & Gordon, E. (2009). Relative contributions of the cerebellar vermis and prefrontal lobe volumes on cognitive function across the adult lifespan. *Neurobiology of aging*, *30*(3), 457-465.

Ramnani, N. (2006). The primate cortico-cerebellar system: anatomy and function. *Nature Reviews Neuroscience*, *7*(7), 511.

Sokunbi, M. O., Staff, R. T., Waiter, G. D., Ahearn, T. S., Fox, H. C., Deary, I. J., Starr, J. M., Whalley, L. J. & Murray, A. D. (2011). Inter-individual Differences in fMRI Entropy Measurements in Old Age. *IEEE Transactions on Biomedical Engineering*, *58*, 3206-3214.

Stoodley, C. J. (2012). The cerebellum and cognition: evidence from functional imaging studies. *The Cerebellum*, *11*(2), 352-365.

Schweizer, T. A., Alexander, M. P., Cusimano, M. & Stuss, D. T. (2007). Fast and efficient visuotemporal attention requires the cerebellum. *Neuropsychologia*, *45*(13), 3068-3074.

Schweizer, T. A., Oriet, C., Meiran, N., Alexander, M. P., Cusimano, M., & Stuss, D. T. (2007). The cerebellum mediates conflict resolution. *Journal of Cognitive Neuroscience*, *19*(12), 1974-1982.

Raz, N., Lindenberger, U., Rodrigue, K. M., Kennedy, K. M,. Head, D., Williamson, A., et al. (2005). Regional brain changes in aging healthy adults: general trends, individual differences and modifiers. *Cerebral Cortex, 15*, 1676–1689.

Raz, N., Schmiedek, F., Rodrigue, K. M., Kennedy, K. M., Lindenberger, U. & Lövdén, M. (2013). Differential brain shrinkage over 6 months shows limited association with cognitive practice. *Brain and cognition*, *82*(2), 171-180.

Stoodley, C. J., Valera, E. M. & Schmahmann, J. D. (2012). Functional topography of the cerebellum for motor and cognitive tasks: an fMRI study. *Neuroimage*, *59*(2), 1560-1570.

Van Veen, V. & Carter, C. S. (2006). Conflict and cognitive control in the brain. *Current Directions in Psychological Science*, *15*, 237-240.

West, R. & Alain, C. (2000). Age-related decline in inhibitory control contributes to the increased Stroop effect observed in older adults. *Psychophysiology*, *37*, 179–189.

INDEX

#

A

B

C

D

E

F

G

H

I

K

L

M

N

O

P

R

S

T

U

V

W